The Wisdom of Exercise Health

Feel Better Than Ever While Protecting Yourself Against a Wide Range of Illnesses

RAMIN MANSHADI, MD

PAGE PUBLISHING, INC.
Conneaut Lake, PA

First originally published by Page Publishing 2021

ISBN 978-1-6624-5582-7 (pbk)
ISBN 978-1-6624-6618-2 (hc)
ISBN 978-1-6624-5583-4 (digital)

Printed in the United States of America

The Wisdom of Exercise Health is a first class book for health care professionals and consumers. This is the second book Dr. Manshadi has written that is not only easy to read and learn from, but packed with personal experiences we can all relate to. I would strongly recommend this book to anyone who wants to learn about heart health and exercise. I thoroughly enjoyed reading it.

Kevin Nagle
Chairman & CEO
Sac Soccer & Entertainment Holdings

Dr. Ramin Manshadi has once again articulated his love of the heart, of health, and of exercise. This compact and informative volume follows his first book, *The Wisdom of Heart Health*, in which he expounded on the marvels of the human cardiovascular system and approaches favorable to its long-term performance. In *The Wisdom of Exercise Health*, he clearly communicates the benefits of exercise, its practical and safe application, and its limitations. He addresses the application of exercise in terms of age, health status, gender, and multiple other potentially complicating factors. Dr. Manshadi provides a valuable narrative tour of the spectrum of cardiovascular disease for the lay reader and the beneficial potential of exercise. All in all, he has produced an important work that will be valuable to all who are interested in the what, why, and how of exercise for health.

Ezra A. Amsterdam, MD
Distinguished Professor, Cardiology and Internal Medicine
Associate Chief (academic affairs), Cardiology
University of California (Davis) School of Medicine
Sacramento, CA

The Wisdom of Exercise Health is a timely reminder of the importance of activity on health and wellbeing. Dr Ramin Manshadi explains the complex relationship activity levels have with many facets of health. He explores scientific evidence and complements it with personal experience, making the book accessible to both health care professionals and exercise enthusiasts alike. Highly recommended to all those looking for a great summary and guide for using exercise as medicine.

Kegan Moneghetti MBBS (hons) FRACP FCSANZ PhD
Clinical Assistant Professor/ Sports Cardiology
Stanford University, Palo Alto, California

The Wisdom of Exercise Health is a poignant tale of why we move our bodies and why movement is an essential cornerstone of health. Artfully blending science with personal experience, Dr. Manshadi provides numerous insights into the relationship between exercise and heart health. This important contribution is truly a "something for everyone" book that I would recommend to all who seek to understand the magic of physical activity.

Aaron L. Baggish MD, F.A.C.C., F.A.C.S.M
Director, Cardiovascular Performance Program
Massachusetts General Hospitlal, Boston, MA, USA
Associate Professor of Medicine, Harvard Medical School
Director, Cardiovascular Performance Program
Massachusetts General Hospital

Dr. Manshadi has produced a highly readable and concise yet thorough review of the many physical and psychological benefits of exercise. Athletes and nonathletes alike will benefit from the practical, evidence-based advice offered here. Dr. Manshadi brings decades of experience as a highly-regarded cardiologist and sports medicine physician to his work. I enjoyed this book and recommend it to anyone seeking to learn more about the benefits of exercise. As Dr. Manshadi writes: "Your health is up to you: Get moving!"

Joseph E. Marine, MD, FACC
Professor of Medicine, Johns Hopkins University School of Medicine

As both a patient of Dr. Manshadi's and as a life-long coach, administrator, and physical educator, I loved this book. The book's purpose is to educate and inspire all of us to take better care of our bodies through exercise—and it succeeds brilliantly. Let's live longer and with more joy."

Dr. Ted Leland
Athletic Director Emeritus Stanford University

The Wisdom of Exercise Health (by Ramin Manshadi, MD, FACC, FSCAI, FAHA, FACP):

As a former professional soccer player and president of *EduKick International Football Academies* since 2001, I must say I was thoroughly impressed by Dr. Manshadi's manuscript, *The Wisdom of Exercise Health*.

It's an interesting, entertaining, and informative read about the overall relevance of exercise as it relates to cardiovascular health, brain health, sleep, stress, and many other factors. I find it particularly useful as a reference for my international student-footballers who participate in our soccer academies worldwide. This will assist them in learning more about the importance (and *wisdom*) of exercise health.

Well done, Dr. Manshadi! As a former teammate of yours in college, I must say that I am very proud of your distinguished career in medicine and in particular this latest achievement, ***The Wisdom of Exercise Health***. Bravo my friend, bravo!

Sincerely,
Joey Bilotta, President and Founder
EduKick International Football Academies

A really informative and well-written book. Dr. Manshadi has gone through the pain of explaining the science behind fitness and good health. I know Ramin well and know how much love and research he has put into writing this book. I have no doubt that Ramin's belief in the Baha'i Faith, his dedication to medical profession, and the love he has for humanity have been a major motivation behind writing this book. This book is a gift for all of us who need professional and scientific advice in order to live a healthier life written in a language that we can all appreciate and understand.

Payam Zamani, Founder, Chairman, and CEO
One Planet, Innovation x Intention

It is with great pleasure to say, "You have knocked it out of the ballpark again!" Congratulations on your upcoming book. Your great talents and efforts have paid off! Your past commitment to help provide defibrillators for schools was awesome and you continually support areas of health and exercise that is beneficial to communities. This book is a definite read for everyone in our overall community and those in youth sports. Thank you, Dr. Manshadi, for your service as a *first responder* and *community leader* investing in our health and in the future of our youth. I am convinced that your accomplishments are well recognized. Best wishes in your future endeavors. I hope to see more of your work in the future.

Michael Merriweather
NFL Three-time Pro-Bowler

Our heart health is a key to living a long and productive life, and Dr. Manshadi brings out his passion as he shows us how exercise plays the starring role.

John Rinehart, President Business Operations, Sacramento Kings

SPECIAL CIRCUMSTANCES: FOR ATHLETES

MOVING FORWARD: YOU ARE IN CHARGE

CONTENTS

ACKNOWLEDGMENTS

My wife, Anissa—thank you for all your support and understanding, for taking care of the family on your own while I spent my limited free time on nights and weekends writing this book on and off for the last four years.

My children, Kian, Kevin, and Katya—I could not have asked God for better kids. You guys always strive to be the best in whatever you do. You are my motivation in life.

My father and mother: my father, who always supported me in life and filled it with important proverbs that added so much to the meaning of life for me; to my mother, who gave of herself through-out her life, from day one going into shock after delivering me, to sac-rificing her arm to protect my head during a bike accident—always encouraging, advising, and supporting me to this day.

My brother Omid, thank you for all your kindhearted support in high school and for having gone through so much hardship in your life and still being able to see the world with kindness as you raised all your four children alone.

Kevin Nagle, I have many acquaintances but very few close solid friends. A man of his word, Kevin has always been there for me. He has been supportive in all of my endeavors and remains a great life consultant.

James Novack, thank you for all your intuitive and outstanding editing skills, spending many hours making sure the book's sentences were written clearly and to the point.

I want to acknowledge all my staff at Manshadi Heart Institute who have worked so effectively and efficiently to help run my office and free up time so I can fulfill my life's goals, such as writing this book. This includes my past and present staff: my administrator; office manager; midlevels Refah Maani, Juanita Zuniga, Rex Ambatali, Trina Eagle, Michelle Abraham, Brooke Fletcher, Rachel Valdez; and all my staff.

In addition, I wish to extend special thanks to the following:

Dr. Ezra Amsterdam: It was because of your love of cardiology that I chose this specialty. You have been my ideal mentor since I was a teenager volunteering to perform EKGs at the UC Davis Medical Center, then conducting research, then learning under you as a fellow. Your genuine enthusiasm for research and patient care helped me become a better physician.

Ralph Brindis and John Harold: past American College of Cardiology presidents whom I have known for many years. Thank you for your sound advice on leadership during my tenure as the president/governor of California Chapter of Cardiology, with an additional thank-you to Ralph for his beautifully written review of my first book, *The Wisdom of Heart Health.*

Norm Lepor, past California ACC president: the predecessor to my tenure in that position, who truly helped our chapter as both leader and role model.

To my colleagues who are super experts in sports cardiology: I have faced some very complicated sports cardiology cases from time to time and feel very fortunate to have these expert friends from whom to seek professional advice: Dr. Aaron Baggish from Harvard, Dr. Matthew Wheeler and Kegan Moneghetti from Stanford, Dr. Thomas G. Allison from Mayo Clinic, and Dr. Michael Emery from Cleveland Clinic.

To all my past soccer coaches who helped me understand the importance of how teamwork and unity are keys to happiness and success in life, *and* can make a championship team, especially my 1982 Cosumnes River College State Championship college team. Many of my teammates ended up playing professional soccer in the United States, Europe, and Mexico—including Cesar Placensia, Ricardo Cobian, Joey Bilotta. In fact, after graduating St. Mary's College and playing professional soccer, Joey Bilotta is now running very successful soccer academies (*Edukick*) throughout the world.

Last but not least, I wish to acknowledge the Baha'i Faith, without which I would have been a lost soul with no purpose in life. From early on, it taught me to be selfless and world-embracing, to love humanity, to respect women, to seek justice, to serve humanity, to strive for excellence, to value and honor science, and seek world peace.

STOP SITTING

Exercise, Sports, and Your Life

CHAPTER 1

YEARNING TO MOVE

The Importance of Exercise

Our bodies are *designed to move.*

As small children, we wanted to move all the time. We simply could not be still! Adults would have the hardest time *trying to keep us from moving,* at the dinner table, in the car. We would not want to sit still at school. It was unnatural to us. We could barely wait for recess to go out and play and run.

Some of us still go out to play, with exercise, sports. Some even compete.

Yet in our modern age, many of us are moving *less than ever before.* Sure, we still love *watching* sports. Competitive athletes moving gracefully, powerfully, skillfully. While we sit on the couch. Sedentary lifestyles have become epidemic—along with chronic ailments like obesity, diabetes, and heart disease—while we reach for coffee or energy drinks to get us through the day. This lifestyle and these epidemics are not unrelated.

And the ailments are occurring despite all our advances in modern medicine.

On the other hand, modern medicine now definitively knows something else: Being physically active benefits most everyone in more ways than we realized. From brisk walks to treadmill runs to professional athletic-level performances—all this yields profound positive effects on our health, energy, happiness, and longevity.

Some of us may chronically *think about* becoming physically active again, but have all kinds of excuses that stop us. We are too out of shape, too tired, too overweight, and too embarrassed about how we would look; do not know how to begin; or worry we might even harm ourselves or cause a heart attack if we suddenly start.

The truth is, to participate in exercise or competitive sports, we need to understand how it can affect our health: both favorably *and potentially negatively* if not done appropriately. That is how we can be good caretakers of the one body we have been granted to carry us through life.

Given all this, it is not an overstatement to say this may be one of the most important books you ever read. One that can improve and even save your life.

Who Is This Book For?

This book addresses readers at every level of physical fitness. This includes the following:

- Sedentary individuals wishing to safely initiate exercise
- People with health issues afraid to start an exercise program
- Athletes already exercising who want to be certain they do so safely or want to "bring it up a notch" (I'm defining *athlete* as anyone actively participating in organized sports teams, such as soccer, football, basketball, etc. or in organized competitions such as running, swimming, cycling marathons, etc.)
- Aging individuals/athletes justifiably concerned with new health-risk factors
- Elite pro athletes and ultramarathoners in top shape who need to learn how to recognize warning symptoms that even they may experience

It is also for *everyone who may still need convincing* that proper exercise can enhance their health, energy, engagement with living, enjoyment, and longevity in ways they may have never before considered.

Medicine Today and the True Miracle Drug

People throughout history have been looking for the miracle drug. That magical elixir as peddled by traveling salesmen back in the Old West and even earlier. Of course, they were charlatans who took advantage of people who, then just as now, desperately wanted to improve their health and lifespan.

Through modern science, we have developed many medications that successfully address *specific ailments* and have been a blessing to many people. Yet these always come with side effects. And in many if not most cases, these drugs address only a particular issue. Not someone's overall health.

Yet more recently, numerous medical studies have shown that the equivalent of a miracle drug does exist right now.

Exercise.

Most people, and frankly most physicians, do not fully appreciate the incredibly far-reaching advantages of a physically active life.

As we will explore together in this book, a broad spectrum of benefits can be enjoyed by the general population, as well elite athletes.

It is important for you to understand all this. Why?

Do Not Expect Doctors to Convince You to Exercise

General practitioner physicians and cardiologists often advise patients to exercise and go on heart-supportive diets as they also perform appropriate testing to diagnose and treat the issues that brought the patient to the office. Yet it is rare that doctors will simply advise exercise and a healthier diet without medication.

That is because they know most patients will not fully commit to change their lifestyle habits.

Yet I have had some that do.

A forty-year-old sedentary male came in with hypertension (high blood pressure), and after determining there were no secondary causes, I discussed diet and exercise and at first started him on medication. Yet he preferred not to take anything. I agreed that if he demonstrated to me that he would improve his diet and increase his exercise sufficiently such that he got to the point he did not need any drugs, we could take him off medication.

He began with slow walking, eventually building up to running a few miles a day, five days a week. He changed his eating habits. When he came back in three months, he had dropped thirty pounds, and his blood pressure was completely normal! He felt far better, had more energy, and more focus! We lowered his medication and continued monitoring and, within another month, stopped the medication entirely.

His blood pressure was perfect.

Yet it is unusual that I have such determined patients who take my advice to aggressively commit to adjusting their diet and exercise regimen.

That is why I am writing this book.

People at *every level* of activity need to truly understand what being physically active can do for their bodies and minds and essentially, how it can change their lives.

In fact, the general public are not the only ones that should appreciate this.

Doctors in Need of "Education" Too

I traveled recently for a medical meeting, where I spoke with one of my medical colleagues. I admitted that even I was having borderline hypertension. My exercise routine had been curtailed after a leg injury, and my healthy diet had lapsed when my schedule became particularly demanding. While I am in favor of medication when needed, I cannot tolerate any of the appropriate medications as they make me fatigued. So I made a choice.

I went 100 percent off caffeine and 90 percent off sodium, tried to lower my stress as much as possible, began doing some minimal exercise, and have since maintained my blood pressure within normal range. But if I deviate even a little, my blood pressure goes up. That is how responsive the body can be! I'm healthy, I'm happy, and I'm doing it naturally without medications and any of the accompanying side effects, I told the doctor.

But the other doctor replied, "Good for you. I've been on medication myself for years now, and this way, I continue to enjoy eating what I want, having my coffee and occasional drinks, and do not spend time exercising. I continue to have my life."

This was from a cardiologist—who should know the benefits of exercise and diet! Yet his is not a singular viewpoint even in the medical community.

Americans have become more and more reliant on drugs as the effortless solution to so many of our medical ills. Many people do not find ways to weave exercise into their schedules. They choose not to spend extra money for healthy foods, instead relying on fast foods because they are quick and cheap.

Why? We like the easy way out, and medicine *appears* to offer that.

Some people prefer not to alter their lifestyle and simply ask, "What drugs do I take?"

But this is not necessarily the best approach for us. *Again, it only addresses the specific medical issue that has surfaced, not our overall health.* Plus, all drugs have some side effects.

Ultimately Up to the Patient

Sometimes I see articles or hear people accusing doctors of only wanting to prescribe the newest drug or other medication as the primary means to treat some disease. For some doctors, this may be true. But the truth is that many patients come in asking or even demanding this of their doctors. The doctor may bring up exercise and diet, but if the patient refuses to take action, then medication is the physician's only recourse. The doctor does not turn the patient away because they will not comply with recommended changes. So the physician treats the patient's condition to the best of their abilities, which often means using drugs to control the symptoms.

What patients need to recognize is that just because the doctor gives them medications, *this does not mean it is the ideal approach* to deal with their condition. As said before, the reality is that most doctors *will* recommend changes to exercise and diet *along* with medication since they know from experience that 90 percent of patients will not comply with the recommendations to alter their lifestyle.

Yet if a patient *is* willing, *is* inclined to be physically active, miraculous results are possible.

Today, I saw a new patient, seventy-eight years old, who was leaner than I am. We did a treadmill stress test on him. I will discuss stress tests in more detail in later chapters. But for now, I will simply say that *how long* a patient is on the treadmill, before the physical stress causes symptoms and the patient must stop, is even more revealing than any changes on the EKG that we conduct at the same time.

I had recently done a stress test on myself and lasted ten minutes, as did a younger, forty-year-old patient of mine that same day. Yet today, this seventy-eight-year-old man lasted the same ten minutes we did! His test results overall were negative (negative is good). He has stayed physically active all his life and even revealed that up until four years ago, he used to bench press two hundred pounds! Most of us do not expect this is even possible for a person in their seventies. Yet he continues to maintain an alert mind and walks with a quick pace, all because of continued activity.

I also had an eighty-two-year-old patient this week who continues to perform all kinds of physical activities on his farm, with no major medical issues.

Both of these individuals reaffirmed my belief that active people are the ones who most often experience a long, high quality of life. They are not feeling old with physical issues and complaining, "Oh, my aches and pains! Sometimes I'd rather just die."

They are healthy enough that they want to live life!

Changing Habits Is Hard and Worth It

Admittedly, habits are hard to change. This applies to both performing physical activities and in the ways we think.

Something must provoke a shift. That can be from a resolute choice we willingly make or from circumstances imposed onto us. The sad fact is that studies show the patients who do change their habits do so most often after some serious medical event has occurred. A heart attack. A stroke. They survive it and say, "Okay, now I'm serious about stopping smoking. I am really going to watch my diet. I will walk and exercise."

Without such a wakeup call, those with a chronic disease state like hypertension or diabetes often would rather take the medication and continue to indulge in life's vices. Yet again, they need to recognize that these medications only address the specific condition *that they know of.* It does not help their overall health or protect them from developing other ailments.

We have all seen people who end up taking a vast array of medications every day. Medications that all have side effects. In fact, sometimes some of those medications are to counter the side effects of their other medications!

Yet they do not realize *how much better they would feel all the time* if they had a healthy lifestyle that included exercise and a better diet rather than just those few moments of pleasure when they indulge a fatty or salty meal or simply lounge around.

They do not know this because they have not yet tried it.

Plus, by committing to exercising and watching our diets, many other possible ailments can be avoided or minimized beyond simply high blood pressure. As you will see in this book, these include cancers, obesity, diabetes, additional risks from heart disease, and even far beyond these.

Happiness

Many of us are willing to work hard at our jobs or at building a business because we anticipate the monetary rewards that can bring. We believe that financial security and abundance will grant us happiness. After all, happiness is the ultimate goal. But what so many are ignoring is the ongoing pleasure and happiness one experiences *when they feel physically great.*

Yes, that takes work and some sacrifice too, as do most good things. But the rewards are profound. And constantly with us.

Why I Am Writing This Book

For all the reasons already mentioned, and for many more that will be revealed in this book, I want to make readers smarter about exercise so

- they better appreciate its incredible benefits;
- they are not afraid to start an exercise program or up the level of activity they already are doing out of fear it could harm themselves (like with a heart attack);
- they find the right physical activities and exercise levels that suit them; and
- athletes at every level, all the way up to competitive and elite professionals, can improve their performance safely and also recognize any symptoms that can be clues that something needs to be addressed.

I will also look at when someone might be well served by having a medical professional who knows sports and exercise medicine advise them how to safely embark on or enhance an exercise program and guide their way. This is not an advertisement for me. My practice is in Stockton, California. Most people reading this book will not come to me for guidance or treatment. But there will likely be others like me that readers can seek out in their geographical area.

In those cases, patients might get what cardiologists call an exercise prescription that is customized for each patient according to their age, health status, physical fitness, etc. Ideally this would come from a sports cardiologist, exercise physiologist, or someone else similarly knowledgeable who knows how to prescribe exercise for different types of patients. You can ask your general practitioner for a referral to such a professional.

This Book Gets You Started

Before you consider whether to seek out a professional's help, this book will elaborate on the advantages of exercise *and* how it can be done safely to avoid causing or worsening any health issues. That way, you will have a far greater understanding of your body, exercise, and what questions to ask if you choose to engage a professional's help.

Lastly, and perhaps most importantly, my intent is to educate so you will be motivated and prepared to follow through on changes that will enhance the rest of your life.

But first, before you read the rest of the book, let us consider its source: me. The next chapter introduces you to my unique background and how it informs both the intent and content of this book.

CHAPTER 2

PHYSICIAN/ATHLETE/AUTHOR

Why I Wrote This Book

I author this book from a rather unique perspective. I am not only a cardiology specialist with a focus on exercise. I have also had a passion for sports throughout my life. Not only as spectator but as an athlete.

I was raised in both Israel and Iran (a pretty unique perspective right there), where there were no opportunities for organized sports when I was young. Instead, I played street soccer. While I cannot claim to have comparable skills, I can point out that the great Pelé of Brazil did not play organized soccer when he was young either. He started in the streets too and became widely regarded as the best player in the world.

Frankly, I think we can steal something precious from young athletes when we plunge them into organized sports *too early*. Many young people have great passion for their sport and simply want to play with all their heart, improving their own unique talents. This early passion can carry them through a lifetime.

There are many benefits to starting sports when young, beyond developing talents. Studies have shown that children involved in sports are less anxious, think more clearly, and have better sleep patterns. Sports also help prevent childhood obesity and diabetes. There are social benefits: learning teamwork and how to strive toward a goal. Sports also teach discipline and, in doing so, helps keep children from getting into trouble. As they get older, individuals that are competitive athletes are less likely to get into drugs as they must remain in top shape. Frankly, they get their high through exercise. They do not need a fake euphoria from doing drugs.

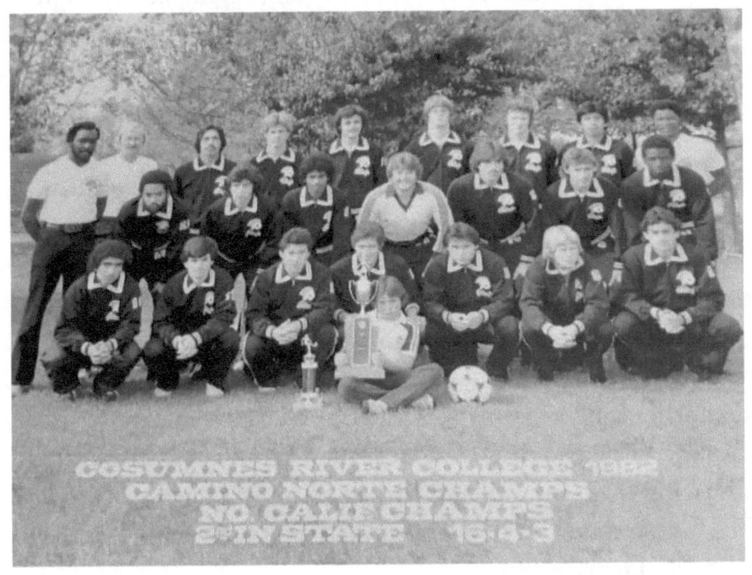

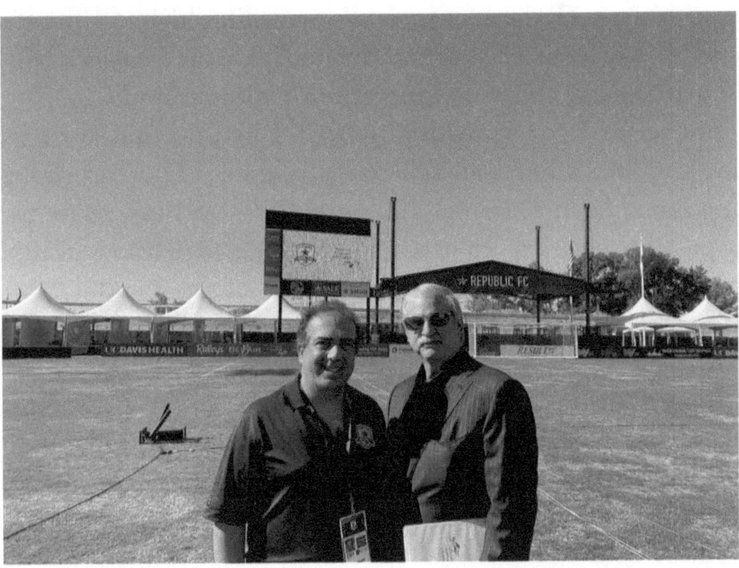

With Kevin Nagle, owner of Sacramento Republic.

California, Here I Come

When I came to live in the United States at the age of twelve, I was introduced to organized soccer and began playing at my high school in Elk Grove, California. Subsequently, I played club soccer for Elk Grove City and traveled to compete against clubs from other cities. To be part of a team was particularly helpful to me, coming from a foreign country to a school that was 99 percent Caucasian. Both myself and my brother assimilated well because of sports. With eighteen players on a team, I immediately had seventeen friends.

Having experience in sports starting from childhood, I then studied physiology at the university level and earned an applied physiology masters before I became a medical doctor. I continued playing soccer competitively in college for two years. But I then realized that I faced another kind of rivalry: competing to make the grades needed to get into medical school. So I took my level of playing down a notch by withdrawing from my college's league team to allow more time for my studies. I played for fun on intramural teams during my last undergrad years at UC Davis.

During this time, I continued to experience the many benefits of being an athlete. All the energy, my enjoying life's highs (without drugs or alcohol). My focus on sports and school gave me a *balance*. My brain was sharp, and my ability to learn seemed without limit.

But when I got to medical school, I had no time for anything but my studies. I gained thirty pounds, and my LDL (bad cholesterol level) jumped from a normal 100 up to 190! So I can relate to what many patients have experienced as I did not always lead a healthy life. Circumstances pushed me from one side of the pendulum (super healthy athlete) to the other (not-so-healthy, stressed-out medical student).

I just want to point out that we are all human beings. Seldom can we always do everything perfectly. I present myself as an example. Even though I knew the benefits of exercise, sometimes life presents us circumstances that push us in the wrong direction.

Once I hit fifty, I had borderline hypertension. Now I am moving the pendulum back the other way because I know if I do not, there will be negative consequences. I also know it is never too late.

From Athlete to Treating Athletes

As a cardiologist with a focus on sports medicine, I have treated patients at every level and every age, from high school competitors to elite athletes, from nine years old to middle-aged to those over one hundred years old. Some athletic and many not. I have had patients who began with me when they were young and others in their eighties whom I told that I would help them make it to a hundred.

Interestingly, I notice the ones who did make it to one hundred had often been active when they were young. One such man had been a judge in the area for many years, who throughout his life would play tennis for an hour during his lunch break, all the way until his eighties. Even though he had stopped playing, all those years of having been active significantly helped him to live longer.

Working with patients of all ages, from all walks of life, with all degrees of athleticism, I have seen great turnarounds. I have assisted and witnessed lives dramatically change for the better. I have *also* seen tragedies occur for people who were not smart about exercising. The reality is anyone can benefit, and anyone can suffer consequences.

That is why *everyone* needs to understand their bodies and exercise.

Treating Professional Athletes

In addition to the typical array of patients seen by a physician, I have also been a doctor for professional sports teams.

I am presently the team cardiologist for the Sacramento Republic professional soccer team. I am also a consultant for all athletes at the University of the Pacific, a private local university. If any of their athletes have cardiovascular issues (arrhythmias, shortness of breath, etc.), they are sent to me. They have a very successful sports program, with young Olympians and potential Olympians coming from all over the world to play for them. Their men's water polo team has been ranked in the top three for the last few years. Their men's soccer team was ranked as high as seventeenth in the nation. Local high schools also send athletes to me. I have also collaborated with the Sacramento Kings basketball team: we did PSAs with two of their players and their coach, raising awareness for the need to place AEDs (automated external defibrillators) in public places.

Likewise, I have been heavily involved in getting AEDs into local high schools for their sports programs since most high schools lack funding for that. I used monies made from my last book and also allied with various companies for donations to purchase these defibrillators for schools.

For the last ten years and continuing, I have coached competitive soccer teams for thirteen- and fifteen-year-olds. One of my teams won the State Cup at the Gold Level three years ago and another won the State Cup Platinum Championships. Both my sons played on these teams, which gave me a way to spend more time with them while also putting together a really good team.

Teaming Up for Health

While it can be valuable for a young person to get involved in any sport, *team sports* offer additional benefits as they connect you to others and teach you to be a team player.

I apply this principle to the leadership role I take in my work. The best way to lead by example is by being a team player. Not to seek personal recognition, but to encourage and empower your team to excel in their needed tasks. This not only helps to motivate and engage everyone involved, it also leads to better patient care.

Take for example my involvement in getting defibrillators donated to high school athletic teams. If another person or organization expresses interest in helping, I wholeheartedly welcome them. We share ideas and resources, collaborating on events to acquire more defibrillators to distribute to more schools. In the end, the schools and students are the beneficiaries, as more athletes can be saved from sudden death by receiving defibrillation.

Frankly, such an attitude helps throughout one's life. Whatever we do, we never do it alone. In a work setting, you communicate with your colleagues or employees in such a way that everyone performs better, promoting unity so the overall approach is successful. Within a family, better results and greater harmony are promoted by working together for goals (even one as mundane as spring cleaning).

Regardless of the scale or size of your group, this approach can likely be applied. Having been elected president of American College of Cardiology, California, I am bringing that same style of participation there. Most presidents have a theme, or legacy, they try to emphasize during their tenure. Fittingly, mine is to raise member awareness regarding exercise, sports, and athletics, and together start initiatives with professional organizations like the NBA, NFL, and MLS.

That is teamwork.

Now I am teaming up with you, the reader, for a similar cause: to bring better health through exercise into your life. By writing this book, I hope to advance attitudes about exercise and improve the health of Americans.

This intention is fully in line with one of my driving forces in life, which has been the philosophies of the Bahá'í Faith. A relatively new religion (established in the nineteenth century), it speaks of the unity of all people, and its teachings promote peace, harmony, and service to humanity. This has fueled my desire to serve others through becoming a physician and now by creating this book.

Now that you know *my* history, let me next tell you about the history of exercise. It is fascinating and may well surprise you. Though much attention today focuses on too many people being sedentary and the resulting ill-health effects, ours is not the first generation or era to be concerned by this.

Not by a long shot.

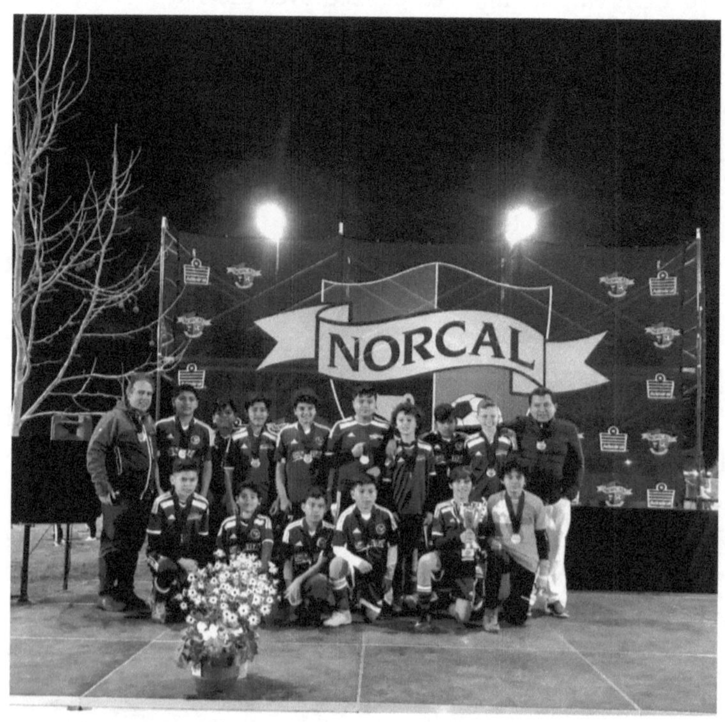

Coaching the state platinum cup championship team, Stockton Storm.

CHAPTER 3

HISTORY OF EXERCISE

Movement throughout the Ages

The history of exercise is intriguing and largely unknown to the public.

If you look far back in human history, you will see there was no problem having sufficient physical activity. Starting eighty thousand to seventy thousand years ago, our primitive caveman ancestors were mostly hunter-gatherers. The men were tracking, chasing, and stalking for days at a time, searching out bigger game and carrying home what they caught. Women would stay active as well, collecting smaller game and gathering plants. Once the men's hunting party returned, there would be feasting for a day or two. Then hunting would commence again.

When the supply of available wild animals shrank in their area, entire villages of people would load up all their possessions to move to another location in the search for fresh supplies of game or for better weather during harsh winters and summers. It was a matter of survival.

Reduction in Physical Activity

Around 10200 BC came the Neolithic period. This was when early technology first was being developed, primarily the usage of Stone Age tools (Neolithic means "new stone.")

Importantly, people began growing plants for food and raising animals for the same purpose rather than only relying on hunting. This allowed people to settle in more permanent villages as they no longer needed to journey in pursuit of game.

As welcome as this change may have been for the tribes, it was the beginning of sedentary lifestyles. While still active with farming and the other daily tasks, they no longer had to hunt nor travel great distances in a constant search for food.

The Dawn of Deliberate Exercise

Persia. It was later, between 4000 and 750 BC, that the Persians became one of the first peoples to realize the importance of exercise. Admittedly, it was designed mainly as an effort to enhance their military. (Other cultures would soon evolve the same strategy.)

All boys became government property after the age of six. They participated in hunting and marching drills, as well as other physical activities to maintain strong bodies so to eventually become good soldiers. At around 2000 BC, Persia was one of the largest empires in the world. Its realm extended all the way east to India and west to North Africa.

But as would repeat throughout history, when one culture's empire became strong and their domain solidified, people began relaxing. Affluence was abundant and corruption occurred at the higher levels. That led to the demise of the Persian empire as they had drifted away from military exercise and mandated that young men be on a path toward soldiering. Eventually, they would be conquered by other countries.

India. Near the same time, a different kind of physical emphasis was finding form in India, one that would play a role there and throughout the world regarding physical health.

India has long had a great focus on spirituality. As a result, there had not been the concentration on physical activity as there was elsewhere. Instead, they created yoga.

Literally meaning "union," yoga was intended to unite the mind, body, and spirit. In fact, most yoga positions and movements imitate those of animals, to help practitioners become harmonized with nature.

China. During this same period in China, it was noticed that sedentary people were more inclined to develop chronic diseases, such as diabetes. So China created the art of kung fu gymnastics. Akin to India's development of yoga, it too imitated the movement of animals. The practice of kung fu increased flexibility and strength and enhanced cardiovascular health to some degree. It was later that kung fu transformed further into a martial art.

Greece. From 2500 to 200 BC, the Greeks were considered the intellectuals of the world. To this day, we still quote their philosophers and teachings (such as those of Socrates and Aristotle).

They realized the importance of body and mind, and their famous physicians, Hippocrates and Galen, promoted exercise for health. Greeks were one of the first to develop both indoor and outdoor palaces called *palestras* that focused on gymnastics and wrestling, as well as other sports, such as javelin throwing. Meanwhile, Sparta, the city-state in northern Greece, learned from the Persians and promoted exercise to help with their military.

Rome. From 200 BC to AD 476, the Romans were focused on a commitment to exercise for military purposes. As needed, they would draft people from ages seventeen to sixty, so men had to remain healthy and fit to be ready for military duty. Recognizing the benefits to overall health as well, they additionally encouraged men and women to exercise independent of the purposes for military duty.

Yet the same plight occurred to the Romans that had with the Persians. As the Empire was successful and lands were conquered, prosperity led to people exercising less and less as they enjoyed a more affluent lifestyle. They became sedentary as servants performed many of the activities they previously had done. Even during that time, a comfortable lifestyle often led to obesity and chronic disease. Individual bodies as well as the military became weaker, allowing the barbarians from the north to come in and take over parts of the Roman Empire. These barbarians were still hunters and fighters and physically stronger. As "barbarians," they destroyed much of the culture that had been built by the Greeks and Romans, leading to the Dark Ages (known also as the early Middle Ages).

Lasting from the late fifth to the tenth centuries AD, this was a more primitive time. All things intellectual remained at a standstill. But exercise became a greater part of daily life again. Not as a health pursuit, but rather, as something again necessary for daily living.

Renaissance and Beyond. After the Dark Ages came the Renaissance. Meaning "rebirth," the Renaissance began in Italy and spread throughout Europe. It brought a return to pursuits of classical learning and humanistic values. Fortunately, it also brought back much of the Greek philosophy, including a focus on the body and intellectual endeavors. Exercise was once again important, but there was no development of it in a structured manner. It remained more as a focus in sports as it had been with the Greeks: running, gymnastics, javelin throwing, etc.

Next came the National Period in Europe as different countries made various contributions to the pursuits of exercise. Germany became one of the first to recommend *structured* exercise, after Napoleon's defeat of them in battle was largely attributed to German physical weakness. Germany began emphasizing the importance of activity and gymnastics.

Sweden divided exercise into three types to serve different purposes: educational gymnastics, military gymnastics, and medical gymnastics. Educational gymnastics was similar to what we today refer to simply as gymnastics. Military gymnastics was intended to prepare soldiers for the rigors of battle. Lastly, medical gymnastics was aimed at people with some medical condition for which they needed to strengthen muscles and joints. This could be applicable to both healing ailments (as one might apply physical therapy), or to preventing future ailments, especially those connected to sedentary lifestyles.

Exercise as Treatment

In England in the mid-1800s, a medical student, Archibald MacLaren, was the first to realize that the cure for people who were tired and fatigued and those with significant stress was physical activity. He devoted his career to studying and teaching the importance of exercise. Additionally, he promoted the *progression* of exercise. That is, someone sedentary should not leap into intense physical challenges such as marathon runs. It was important that the individual progressively increase their exercise regimen over time.

Physical Activity in the United States

During America's colonial period of 1700 to 1776, there had been no promotion of exercise or physical activity for its own sake. Most inhabitants were actively involved in hunting for game or working the earth for farming as people established homesteads on undeveloped lands. The culture returned to a Neolithic agriculture lifestyle.

Yet as the United States developed, European cultures had a greater influence. Immigrants from England, Germany, and Sweden began to focus again on physical activities. Interestingly, Ben Franklin was one of those who emphasized fitness. Later, Thomas Jefferson encouraged everyone to exercise at least two hours a day (far beyond today's suggested minimum of thirty minutes of brisk walking, five days a week). He commented, "If the body be feeble, the mind will not be strong."

In the 1800s, educator and author Catharine Beecher promoted calisthenics and fitness, especially for women. The activities that she designed were very similar to what later became known as aerobics.

The post-Civil War period from 1865 to 1900 was a time of industrialization in the United States, with more people living in urban areas. Of course, once one leaves a rural setting, there is less emphasis on physical activity. Chronic ailments such as cardiovascular disease, diabetes, and cancers increased as a result of this decrease in physical activity.

At the start of the twentieth century (1901 to 1909), we had perhaps the most fit president ever to hold that office, Theodore Roosevelt. Though he suffered from debilitating asthma as a child, he overcame his condition through a commitment to rigorous physical activity, particularly in the outdoors. For that reason, he was a lifelong advocate of exercise, embracing the emphasis on its importance in Greek philosophy. Anecdotally, I have observed that among my patients, many of the healthiest have been avid hikers.

Yet when the United States entered into World War I in 1917, one-third of those drafted for the military were unfit. That led to serious questions about how fit we were as a nation. Physical fitness was suddenly given great emphasis once again.

However, after the war was won, everyone relaxed in these efforts. The nation felt relieved, and habits gave way to pleasures and partying as society became affluent. The Roaring Twenties was born. Plus, increasing numbers of people were living in cities, and exercise again held less significance in society.

World War II

After Pearl Harbor was bombed in 1941, it was found that half of military draftees were unfit (contrast with one-third of unfit draftees in World War I). A doctor named Thomas Cureton at the University of Illinois became one of the first to advocate research to better understand exercise through scientific methods. He studied what kind of exercise is important, how much is needed, etc.

This time after the war ended, exercise did not fall into the background as far as it had after the First World War.

Television prevented this in part, with the advent of *The Jack LaLanne Show*, an exercise TV program that aired from 1951 to 1985. Considered the father of fitness, Jack LaLanne originated a variety of types of exercise, introduced new kinds of exercise equipment, and created a series of health clubs bearing his name. With help from this new media of television, he was able to promote an exercise-centered lifestyle again.

Children Included Too

In 1950s, Hans Kraus, MD, and Ruth P. Hirschland published results of a study that would eventually introduce minimum muscular fitness standards for children. The research (encompassing 4,264 American and 2,870 European children) evaluated both strength and flexibility of trunk and leg muscles. It found that nearly 60 percent of American children failed this test (actual numbers were 57.9 percent American children failed, while only 8.7 percent of the European children did). The conclusion was that industrial modernization in America had led to much lower overall levels of physical activity. This led to President Dwight D. Eisenhower establishing the President's Council on Youth Fitness to produce programs for getting our children fit.

During the 1950s, many health organizations formed, including the American Heart Association, the American Medical Association, the California American Medical Association (for which I am a delegate), along with the American College of Sports Medicine, which has become one of the premier authorities in exercise medicine in the United States.

This advocacy continued, and in the early 1960s, John F. Kennedy said, "Physical fitness is the basis for all other forms of excellence." During this same period, Dr. Ken Cooper became the first person to promote exercise not only for strengthening and remedying ailments but also for *preventing* them. He introduced a new approach to exercise called *aerobics* and has been credited with getting more people to exercise than anyone else in history.

Exercise Today

These more recent developments have led us to our present state of greater awareness among doctors and the general populace regarding exercise. Health clubs exist in most major cities. Exercise equipment can be found in many apartment and condo buildings, and even private homes. Jogging and running have become popular pastimes.

Individuals exercise today for various reasons. Fortunately, health remains a primary motivator as people feel better and enjoy increased energy with regular exercise. Plus, it improves appearance as it can help people stay trimmer and even look younger.

CHAPTER 4

MEN AND WOMEN EQUAL AT LAST

Women's Heart Health at Risk

I include this very short chapter because I want to be certain this is not missed in your reading. It addresses one more piece of history that must be recognized.

As described in the last chapter, throughout most of our evolution, physical activity has been essential to everyday life, whether it be as hunters, farmers, or builders.

It was not until we began relying on agriculture and raising animals for food (no longer living as hunter-gatherers) that this began to change for many populations. Technological advancements have reduced the need for physical activity even further.

During more recent decades in the United States and elsewhere, we have become increasingly sedentary. Many occupations have evolved into literally sitting all day at a computer. Recreation has been reduced to sitting long hours in front of a television or, again, at a computer. With food abundant in most western societies, people are eating more than in times past.

And we are definitely seeing the effects of this.

Heart disease, heart attacks and strokes, obesity, diabetes, weaker bones and muscles, hormonal imbalances, inflammation, increases in depression and anxiety are all consequences of our inactivity.

This is true for both sexes, *including heart disease, which, in more recent times, has become an increasing concern for women.*

Historically, the focus on heart disease has been mostly with men. It simply did not appear as commonly in women. Because of their hormones, women are protected longer from heart disease. On average, such ailments do not appear until ten to fifteen years later than in men. In the past, before women were commonly living into their fifties, when heart disease was more prone to occur, a woman likely would have died from other causes first. It was not apparent that women could suffer heart attacks or strokes as did men.

Being a man provides a higher risk for having heart disease *primarily because the onset of such illness occurs earlier* than in women. Yet risks of heart disease for men and women become essentially equal after a certain age. This is why there has been much more attention regarding heart disease and women in recent decades, since now we enjoy more longevity. With people living longer, the negative effects of heart disease and our sedentary lifestyles are becoming glaringly obvious for everyone.

BENEFITS OF EXERCISE

Understanding How Your Body Functions

CHAPTER 5

EXERCISE AND CARDIOVASCULAR HEALTH

While these next four chapters address some major benefits from exercise, additional chapters will allude to others as well.

Our bodies are truly amazing.

This is certainly the case whenever we are physically active or exercising, be it walking briskly, jogging, competing in sports, or participating in ultramarathons.

It should be noted that *physical activity* and *exercise* are words used interchangeably in everyday language. But when speaking with physicians, these are scientific terms with specific meanings.

Physical activity (called PA for short) is any body movement produced by our (skeletal) muscles that causes a caloric expenditure.

Exercise is also body movement, but a *planned* type of physical activity done in a manner to promote physical fitness. It qualifies as exercise even if just a brisk walk for ten minutes (minimum). Ideally, thirty minutes or more at one time is preferred, but even ten minutes in three portions meets the criteria for exercise.

Exercising or competing can place great demands on the body, though most of us are unaware how the body coordinates so many functions simultaneously to meet that demand. Yet this awareness will help us appreciate the magnificence of our physical being, as well as potential risks that such activities can place on our body. Hopefully, this will also motivate us to take better care of it!

In no area is this truer than in our cardiovascular system, by which the blood travels throughout the body. There is a fascinating cyclical arrangement between our circulatory system and exercise: A healthy cardiovascular system improves our performance, and exercise improves our cardiovascular system.

Talk about win-win.

Blood Transportation

The main function of our heart and blood vessels is to supply oxygen to tissues throughout our body. This oxygen travels in the hemoglobin and red blood cells of the blood, which circulates through over *sixty thousand miles* of blood vessels in the body, pumped by the heart that beats more than one hundred thousand times a day.

Just thinking about that is stunning.

Yet exercise dramatically increases the demand for oxygen to certain areas of our body. The heart works harder to increase the cardiac output and deliver more blood and oxygen to these tissues. This increase is determined by the *stroke volume* (amount of blood pumped during each heartbeat) and the *heart rate* (number of beats per minute).

As we exercise, our body *shifts where it sends the blood* to meet needed demands. More flows to the active muscles and the skin (to dissipate heat so we do not overheat). Some other areas receive *less* blood—such as the gastrointestinal tract, liver, kidneys—as they do not need as much oxygen since they are not utilized during exercise.

Now, how much our cardiovascular system needs to adjust its output will depend on several factors:

- How intense the exercise (the more intense, the greater oxygen demand)
- Duration (is it five minutes or thirty minutes or one hour)
- How much muscle mass is being utilized (if jogging, it is mostly leg muscles; if rowing, more muscles are exerting).

So what happens at the onset of exercise?

How the Active Body Functions

As said, one goal of the cardiovascular system is to increase blood flow to the most active skeletal muscles. You can imagine this would be complex, yet the body does it automatically. We do not even think about it.

Here is why: Our body uses two types of nerve systems. The first is the *autonomic nervous system*. It controls certain body functions without any effort by our higher brain function, such as our heartbeat and blood flow, as well as breathing and digestion.

There is also the *somatic nervous system*. This is where the brain directs the voluntary control of the skeletal muscles if we want to run, walk, climb, swim, etc.

Autonomic Nervous System

Within the autonomic nervous system, there are two divisions: the *sympathetic nervous system* that speeds things up and the *parasympathetic nervous system* that slows things down.

Let me explain.

When you exercise, the sympathetic system is activated. It causes the heart to squeeze harder (increasing the volume of blood pumped with each beat) and raises the heart rate. This increases oxygen delivery to the organs in need. Along with other body responses that we will discuss, this is sometimes called the fight-or-flight response. It is the same reaction that enabled our ancient ancestors either to fight or run away when confronted with a dangerous animal or formidable opponent. That same autonomic response continues in us today when we are physically active, including when facing off against sports competitors rather than a saber-tooth tiger.

On the other hand, the parasympathetic nervous system tends to undo the sympathetic system responses *after* a stressful situation, so the body can relax, rest, or assimilate food. It slows the heart and respiration, dilates blood vessels (lowering blood pressure), constricts the pupils, increases urine output, and stimulates digestion.

Sympathetic Nervous System and Physical Activity

Other changes occur in your body as well during exercise.

In addition to the cited increases in heart rate and volume, the *systolic blood pressure* also goes up. This is the upper larger number in the blood pressure measurement and represents the amount of pressure on blood vessels when the heart pumps blood into the body.

The heart is already pumping more strongly to move more oxygen-carrying blood to where it is needed. Arteries will also constrict, raising their resistance to blood flow (called peripheral resistance) that helps *push blood* through the blood vessels. Together, they deliver more oxygen to the tissues.

But it should be noted that the heart, which is already exerting more during exercise, also has to work harder because it is pumping against this increased (systolic) blood pressure. Both these factors determine how much stress the heart experiences during exercise, something we will consider later in the book in regard to advice about how best to approach exercise at all levels of exercise and competition.

(Meanwhile, the diastolic blood pressure stays the same or drops slightly by about 10. The diastolic pressure is the lower, smaller number in the blood pressure measurement and represents the pressure in the arteries when the heart rests between beats.)

During exercise, blood flow *back to the heart* (called *venous return*) is stronger too. That is because skeletal muscles compress the venous vessels to increase this flow, while one-way valves in the peripheral veins (especially in arms and legs) guide flow away from the muscle and back toward the heart.

More Changes Occur Simultaneously

When we put our bodies under physiological stress during exercise, it causes other interactions in the body as well.

Our sympathetic nervous system enhances our brain's ability to get feedback from our senses (such as sight and hearing), from our skeletal muscles, and from our *baroreflex receptors*, which gauge the pressure in our main blood vessels that travel to the body, as well as our carotid artery that goes to the brain. Those receptors inform the brain if there is too much pressure, and it needs to reduce by dilating (widening) blood vessels so we do not have a stroke. They also signal if there is too little pressure so that it can be increased so we do not pass out.

In addition, the sympathetic system engages other body functions, such as dilating (expanding) the lung's bronchioles to bring more air into the lungs and increase oxygenation of the blood, stimulating adrenal glands to release performance-enhancing hormones, and more.

As you can see, the level of sophistication in the body is dazzling.

Now let us dive a little deeper into these two important issues during exercise: blood *pressure* and blood *flow*.

Changes in Blood Pressure

Typically, during the first fifteen minutes of exercise, the systolic blood pressure (pressure during the heart's contraction) should rise. However, the diastolic pressure (pressure when the heart relaxes to refill) should either not change or may drop a little. At the same time, the baroreflex receptors that I mentioned (in the aorta and the carotid arteries) will tell the brain if the blood pressure is going *too high*, which will then cause the vessels to dilate to lower it. Systolic blood pressure can rise to 180 to 200 when doing very aggressive exercise. But it should not go higher as that can cause issues, including a bloody nose or possibly stroke.

In fact, there is another way the body adjusts itself so blood pressure does not go too high called *cardiovascular drift*. The heart rate goes up, but the stroke volume (amount of blood pumped during each heartbeat) goes down, and this lowers the blood pressure. The cardiac output still remains higher to meet the muscles' increased oxygen demands for the exercise because the heart rate goes up, even if the amount of blood pumped by each heartbeat is less.

During physical activity, while you may only be aware of how fast you are moving, if you are out of breath, or if your body feels at ease or aches, your body is dynamically adjusting and compensating to allow you to safely perform at your best.

Again, as always, amazing.

It is worth noting that systolic blood pressure (the higher number) *should never drop* during physical activity, though it should *flatten out* (remain constant at some maximum number) at peak exercise. If it *drops* during exercise, that signifies issues with the heart. In fact, when we do treadmill stress tests on patients in our office, one of the problem indicators we check for is whether the systolic blood pressure lowers when a patient is exercising. That usually means they have three vessel blockages. (There are three main arteries connecting to the heart, and when we see arterial disease, that means they have significant blockages in all three). Because the heart itself is not getting sufficient oxygen (since it receives insufficient blood due to blockages), the heart does not operate properly, and the blood pressure drops.

Changes in Blood Flow

So how much does blood flow distribution change during exercise?

Answer: an impressive amount.

Under normal circumstances, when not exercising, the *skeletal muscles* get 18 to 20 percent of all the circulating blood. Yet during exercise, 85 percent of blood circulation flows to the active muscles. To put that in measurable numbers, the normal flow of blood to involved skeletal muscles can go from sixteen milliliters (ml) per minute during periods of nonexercise to four thousand milliliters per minute during intense physical activity!

You might think you would pass out when this occurs (as less blood could be available to the brain and other organs), but you must realize that when you exercise, at most 50 percent of the skeletal muscles are typically active. So in reality, blood flow increases *to many areas* during physical activity.

This includes increases in flow to the coronary arteries (for the heart muscle to function) and respiratory arteries (for the lungs to oxygenate blood). That is why if there is coronary artery disease such as blockages, people start having symptoms when exercising. Physical activity raises the demand for oxygen-carrying blood *to the heart muscle* so it can operate at higher, more stressful levels. But if the heart *does not receive* sufficient amounts due to a blockage, the heart muscle will begin aching. That is a symptom commonly noticed by lay people if they have coronary artery disease. But that indicator does not require there to be heavy exercise. I have patients coming in who report they were mowing their lawn when they felt tightness in their chest. I almost do not need to perform further testing to know they have a blockage. In fact, 90 percent of diagnosing blockages is done by learning the patient's history, with the other 10 percent sourcing from their exam and lab work.

So how much does blood flow increase to the heart and lungs during exercise?

Normal coronary blood flow is 250 milliliters per minute, but during physical activity, it can rise to 1,000 milliliters per minute. Blood flow to the lungs will depend on the necessary surge in breathing. Normally, respiratory blood flow rises 10 to 15 percent. (Note that respiratory flow not only involves the lungs but also the intercostal muscles that help the lungs expand and contract in order to breathe.)

VO2 Max

Let me introduce a concept that will be mentioned several times in this book. *VO_2 max* is the measurement of total oxygen uptake: the maximum amount of oxygen an individual's body can utilize during exercise (V = rate, and O_2 = oxygen). Basically, this reflects the cardiovascular system's ability to supply oxygen to the working skeletal muscles during intense physical activity. It tells how efficient your system is. Some people use this to determine one's overall fitness.

To get an exact measurement requires a cardiopulmonary exam, in which the patient wears an oxygen face mask while taking a treadmill stress test. It measures your oxygen exchange with carbon dioxide, which determines your VO_2 max. That number is the best signifier of how stressed your body is during exercise. It also tells us when you change from aerobic to anaerobic supplying energy to the tissues. VO_2 max is the rate of oxygen that your body utilizes during exercise. It is measured in ml/kg/minutes. The higher it is, the better you can perform.

This test is usually reserved for elite athletes (plus those with heart failure or valve disease) to see how well their system is working. Most private practice cardiologists do not have the equipment for this test, and patients are sent to university facilities for testing.

Flow to Skin

It may surprise readers to learn that the largest organ in the body is the skin. For a person at rest, blood flow to their skin is 200 to 500 ml/minute. But if they are in an environment that is already hot and they are exercising, the arteries around the skin have to open up in order to cool off the body. Blood flow can rise to 3,500 to 4,000 ml/minute! That is why exercising in extreme temperatures can put a significant strain on your heart. When you exercise and the ambient temperature is very hot, the skin and the muscles have to compete for that blood flow. That makes the heart work harder and can bring risks if the heart already has medical issues.

Practical advice is to avoid exercising during the hottest part of the day since the body has to work harder, not only to cool off the body by vessel dilating (expanding) the arteries near the skin but also because the skeletal muscles may be starving since they also need additional oxygen from the blood for their increased physical activity, and more is going instead to the skin to make sure the body does not overheat.

Flow to the Brain

At rest, the normal cerebral blood flow is 12 to 15 percent of the total flow. Exercise significantly increases brain blood flow to the brain.

Blood to Splanchnic Organs

Splanchnic organs are those in the gastrointestinal tract.

These include the liver, pancreas, spleen, stomach, and intestines. When we are at rest, 25 percent of the total blood flow goes to these organs. But during exercise, this *reduces*—from 1,500 ml/minute to 350 ml/minute.

This is why it is not a good idea to eat before exercise.

Normally, extra blood flow is diverted to the digestive organs after a meal. But during exercise, these organs get *even less* blood flow/oxygen than normal. The result is food may not digest well, and you can get nauseous. It should be noted that blood flow to the kidneys drops as well during exercise.

Prolonged Aerobic Exercise

Until this point, I have been describing our body's internal actions during general exercise.

- But how does our body respond differently to prolonged exercise, activity that typically lasts over an hour?
- And what factors determine why some people tire really quickly, while others can continue much longer?

There are several variables that will affect any individual's performance:

- The level of the exercise (Are they just walking or exerting intensely?)
- Their muscle mass (Leaner muscle performs the same tasks with less effort; plus, lean muscles have a better vascular system to deliver oxygen more efficiently.)
- The environmental conditions where the exercise is taking place (hot, humid setting; cold climate; comfortable midseventies degrees environment with low humidity)

Another obvious factor relates to how fit you are: Have you been participating in an exercise regimen?

Yet there are other aspects over which you have no control: What is your genetic makeup? Are you naturally athletic? Do you have fast twitch muscles or slow twitch muscles? (Muscle fibers either respond fast or more slowly to movement. Sprinters and high jumpers tend to have fast fiber muscles, while long-distance runners are better served by slow fiber muscles.) Or perhaps you might be a slow metabolizer. Or genetically have nonlean, nonefficient muscles?

All these factors are at play as our bodies respond to prolonged exercises.

Male and Female Differences

The responses within men's and women's bodies to exercise is much the same. For instance, the variations in blood flow going to different body areas are similar.

But there are differences.

Men have greater amounts of lean muscle, and leaner muscle can perform the same tasks with less effort. Plus, lean muscles have a better vascular system to deliver oxygen more efficiently. Men also have a larger heart size, which can pump more blood volume.

In partial compensation for their smaller hearts, as physical activity increases and oxygen demand goes up, female bodies raise their heart rate to increase blood flow. So the resulting overall blood flow is the same with men and women due to women's heart rates usually going higher than men's during exercise of the same intensity.

But men's bodies still have some other advantages. To some degree, a man's systolic blood pressure is able to rise a little higher than a woman's. Plus, men's bodies have greater oxygen-carrying capacity because they have more red blood cells and hemoglobin. Red blood cells are such an important factor in sports that some Olympic doping scandals involved competitors taking shots of Procrit so their bodies produce more red blood cells.

The result of these many factors is that the VO_2 max (the body's ability to transport oxygen to muscles) remains 40 to 60 percent higher for men, helping to explain why men tend to have greater capacity in exercise performance than women.

Cardiovascular Response and Aging

In general, athletic performance is highest when we are younger. Most of us know this, but how many of us understand why? It is because our body responds differently to exercise as we age.

For instance, the stroke volume (capacity to pump blood volume) drops because the force of our heart muscle contractions decreases. This is due to the heart muscle walls becoming stiffer, which not only reduces the strength of contractions, but also diminishes the heart's ability to relax in between. Since the heart fills with blood while it relaxes between beats, if the heart cannot relax well, it is unable to fill the heart with as much blood volume to pump out. So overall blood flow drops as we age.

Another factor is that oxygen is not taken up as well by the muscles as there is less lean muscle as we get older (again, lean muscle is more efficient in utilizing oxygen).

Plus, as we grow older, the resting *systolic* blood pressure goes up, so the heart has to work harder. Regardless of whether you are young or old, the *degree* to which systolic blood pressure can rise remains the same. But if, as we age, we start with a resting systolic about 20 milliliters higher, that systolic pressure during exercise ends up higher too (usually about 15 milliliters higher). As a result, blood pressure can be expected to rise during exercise for older people to 220, but should not go above 200 for young people.

Alternatively, *diastolic* blood pressure typically remains about the same level when we exercise (it should not go up), though it can rise a little in older people.

In addition, the total peripheral resistance (resistance of arteries to flow of blood) is higher as we age because arteries become less elastic. They do not dilate (widen to allow more blood flow) as easily, and this makes the heart work harder to pump the blood to tissues.

There is also less oxygen going to the muscles because the body generates fewer red blood cells as we age. There are also fewer capillaries (smallest blood vessels from which tissues extract oxygen) in muscle fibers.

Adding to this, the mitochondrial mass is also diminished. The mitochondria are responsible for cell metabolism and providing energy.

Plus, our body's ability to raise its heart rate decreases as we get older. This is readily apparent in our offices as we conduct stress tests on individuals as they get older. We witness that their bodies are not capable of reaching the same heart rates as they had previously. In fact, the maximum heart rate one can achieve can generally be calculated as 220 minus your age. The older you are, the smaller that number.

That is important because higher heart rates facilitate performance during exercise.

As a result, the VO_2 max (ability to deliver oxygen to tissues) is lower in older people. Even though the systolic blood pressure is higher than it is for younger individuals, the lower heart rate has a greater diminishing effect on the VO_2 max.

In fact, after the age of thirty, your VO_2 max generally drops 10 percent per decade. So it is a bigger challenge to achieve the same results you once did. Clearly this gives advantages to the young.

However, older people *can increase their VO_2 max* by about 20 percent in six months through endurance training. If you compare someone young and sedentary with someone who is old but exercises regularly, their exercise capacities would be about the same.

This means that you can basically slow your physiological age with exercise.

In Summary, Our Bodies Are Astonishingly Complex

Now that we have explored the variety of changes that occur in the body when physically active, you can better appreciate the extraordinary gift that your body provides to enhance performance *and* protect your health. From increasing heart rate and stroke volume, to intensifying blood flow and oxygen intake, to releasing hormones that improve physical movement, to boosting the brain's ability to obtain feedback from skeletal muscles and from baroreflex receptors to adjust blood pressure to guard against stroke and keep us from passing out, to elevating our lung bronchiole's ability to increase oxygenation, and much more.

This is why we want people to start slowly in a proper manner as they get into exercise. There is stress associated with so many changes occurring in our body as it tries to amplify our performance. If one is sedentary and suddenly starts playing soccer or running sprints, it places great demand on the body. Sometimes, too much.

Further, knowing that our bodies are so complex will hopefully help motivate us to respect our physical being and take the actions recommended in this book to keep it healthy.

As you can also see, even with all our modern advances, medications cannot completely compensate for us not taking good care of our precious body. The results will never be the same. Plus, no medication is perfect. There are always side effects. Our body *is designed* to operate at and feel its best *through exercise and good diet.* Both are far superior to any medication.

Bottom line: You will discover how much we can improve not only athletic performance but also your overall well-being. When your body is feeling great, it has a stunning positive effect on your outlook on life and happiness.

Let us now look at just a few of the well-proven positive effects that exercise has on our body.

CHAPTER 6

EXERCISE AND SLEEP AND STRESS

Sleep is important.

In fact, critically important.

We hear this constantly today. From doctors. Television news. Newspapers and magazines. The Internet. So why all this current focus?

Because poor sleep is an epidemic today, with seventy million people in the United States estimated to suffer from sleep disorders.

Many of the more positive benefits of good sleep are well-known: having sufficient energy and alertness, the ability to handle life's challenges, the ability to focus, improves memory, etc.

Yet most people do not *really* appreciate the many benefits to sleep or grasp the price we pay when we do not get enough. Especially when this becomes a habit.

Secrets of Sleep

Many processes occur while we sleep. The heart rate and blood pressure fluctuate during sleep, which helps promote cardiovascular health. Cells and tissues are repaired due to an increase in growth hormones released during slumber. Other hormones released during sleep promote a healthy immune system to fight off infections. There is also a hormone released (from fat cells) called leptin that helps to suppress appetite. If too little leptin is released due to insufficient sleep, it causes

56

your brain to perceive that you do not have enough energy to meet your needs, so your brain tells the body that you are hungry. (Alternatively, there is also a hormone called ghrelin that *increases* appetite. But sufficient sleep reduces the release of this hormone.)

Effects of Exercise on Sleep for Insomniacs

A 2013 study out of Northwestern University and published in the *Journal of Clinical Medicine* looked at patients over the age of fifty-five with chronic insomnia. Half of the patients in the trial continued their sedentary lifestyles, while the other half participated in the minimal recommended exercise (150 minutes per week).

For the first four months, these chronic insomnia patients did not gain immediate benefits from the exercise. But beginning just after that initial four-month period, they found that those individuals exercising were getting an hour more of sleep per night compared to the sedentary patients.

While the answers may be a bit more complex than what was shown by this research, other studies have shown that just ten minutes of exercise per day by itself improves nighttime sleeping. I believe that people with chronic insomnia who exercise change their hormonal release patterns to correct the negative neuro-hormonal effects they have developed over time.

Noninsomniacs Benefit Too

Exercise can also improve sleep of those not suffering from insomnia.

Another study, published in the *Journal of Mental Health and Physical Activity*, looked at 2,600 patients, both male and female, ages eighteen through eighty-five, a broader age range than simply over fifty-five. This included a wide variety of people beyond those with chronic insomnia. They found that among those who did the minimum 150 minutes of exercise per week, 65 percent had improvement in their sleep quality. On top of that, they found that 65 percent of them had less leg cramps compared to their condition prior to exercising.

So what is the mechanism by which exercise improves sleep in general?

That answer is not fully known. But it is believed that when you exercise, you increase your body heat, especially if that activity occurs in the afternoon or early evening. Then later when the body heat cools off, the cooling promotes sleep.

So should you exercise in the evening?

It has long been believed that strenuous exercise in the late evening can actually make it harder to get to sleep. Consensus now appears to be that brisk walking—rather than, perhaps, running—in the evening can better help you fall asleep quicker. Another advantage to exercise is that it can also reset the body's circadian rhythm, our internal clock that affects our body's sleep/wake cycle.

How Much Sleep Is Needed?

This varies from person to person, but some general ranges have been found to correlate with different age groups:

- Preschool ages three to five: *ten to thirteen hours*
- School-aged children from six to thirteen: *nine to eleven hours*
- Teenager ages fourteen to seventeen: *eight to ten hours*
- Young adults eighteen through twenty-five: *seven to nine hours*
- Ages twenty-six to sixty-four: *seven to nine hours*
- Older adults over sixty-five: *seven to eight hours*

Interestingly, you will find people at each of these ages who say they do not need that many hours of sleep. But you will *also* find many of those people get tired, need coffee, or some kind of sugar supplement to help them through the day, or simply complain of being bored or lacking passion, etc.

Do Not Wait to Start

One takeaway from this is to start an exercise program early on after you begin noticing your sleep duration reducing. In fact, such a proactive stance is true for many, if not most, medical conditions. With cancer, the earlier you detect and begin treatment, the better. Similarly, the sooner you recognize a pattern of chronic anxiety and deal with that, the better, as the neurohormonal changes that have occurred in the brain can begin reversing more easily.

If you allow your insomnia to become chronic, it may take longer to achieve the benefits offered by adding exercise into your life. So do not become discouraged if adding an exercise regimen does not immediately improve your sleep. It will simply take longer with chronic insomnia.

Further Benefits

It has been found that not only can exercise increase the *duration* of sleep, exercise in general can cause you to *fall asleep faster* as well. Exercise helps reduce stress, and people under stress often have difficulty drifting off into sleep as their minds fixate on whatever life issues are causing their worry.

Another benefit: Exercise can also enhance *the quality* of sleep. It allows you to have more time in restorative *REM* sleep and *slow-wave sleep* (SWS). Though less often addressed, SWS is a sleep phase that allows the body and mind to rebuild itself each night. It is during this time that most human growth hormones (HGH) are secreted to repair body tissues and promote healthy metabolism. Additionally, some researchers believe SWS has an important function in maintaining brain health.

Interestingly, just as some studies have shown that only ten minutes of daily exercise by itself can improve nighttime sleeping, that same amount of exercise has also been shown to improve restless leg syndrome (cramps in your legs at night) and sleep apnea.

Most of us do not get the amount of sleep that allows our bodies to function at their best. Older adults may complain of being tired and think it is simply due to aging. Truthfully, most of us (at any age) do not appreciate how much better, happier, more energetic, and more passionate we could feel if we gave our bodies what they needed. Often, we take better care of our automobiles (with oil changes, service, quality gasoline) than our own bodies!

That is pretty stunning.

Stress

Along with sleep, a great deal of attention is paid to stress in our society as demanding fast-paced lives shower emotional and mental stress upon people of all ages.

To fully understand what stress does, we must appreciate that it produces a *physical reaction* in the body. Most apparent, it causes a fight-or-flight response. This automatic reaction traces back to our ancestors, who, when confronted with intense danger (as in the form of an attacking animal), had two options: fight or flight (run away). The body would immediately prepare them for either action, releasing an array of hormones to raise heart rate and blood pressure, strengthen muscles, increase energy levels, and even suppress fear so they could fight if necessary. A remarkable body mechanism to help humans deal with extreme challenges sometimes faced in the past.

Today, however, most of us do not face life-and-death issues with anywhere near the same frequency or intensity. But this physical response still occurs. Today, different issues trigger stress. Those can range from losing your car keys when you need to race to an important meeting, to discovering your bank account overdrawn, to facing a rude boss or a challenging school exam, or difficulties in love and relationships. Stress can come from confronting our own health issues or those facing loved ones.

While the circumstances may not be as immediately life-threatening, our body still responds by releasing the same hormones, potentially causing all kinds of havoc.

Types of Stress

From the medical point of view, there are three kinds of stress:

- Acute stress
- Episodic acute stress
- Chronic stress

Acute stress is the type most commonly noticed by people. It can arise from temporary challenges like the frantic search for car keys, a job interview, giving a speech, taking an exam, dealing with a school bully, facing any kind of taxing situation. We may experience a racing heart, shortness of breath, irritability, tension, headache, stomachache or heartburn, and other symptoms. Acute stress typically sources from pressures caused by recent or current events or something anticipated to occur in the near future. Effects are usually short-lived.

Episodic acute stress is when such stress occurs frequently during the day or week. In those cases, the effect can be cumulative. If these circumstances and our reactions to them are not dealt with, it can lead to hypertension, among other ailments.

Then there is *chronic stress*. This is where the stress is long-lasting, for weeks to months, with ongoing anxiety, tension, depression, and fatigue. The fight-or-flight stress hormones are continually released into the body. It can become exceedingly hard on you both emotionally and physically, resulting in severe anxiety and depression and even suppression of the immune system. Furthermore, this type of stress can negatively affect the inner lining of the arteries, making them unstable and sticky, such that fat cells/plaque can easily adhere to them. A negative cascade of events can ensue, causing inflammation that in turn causes more damage to the endothelium (artery inner lining), such that blockages can develop to cause heart disease and possible heart attacks.

Fortunately, people who exercise regularly can defend against the effects of these stresses.

From a cardiovascular viewpoint, there can be dramatic differences between those who are sedentary and those who are more active.

Inactive people tend to have less healthy blood vessels that are stiffer. In those cases, the body's release of stress hormones constricts the blood vessel and increases blood pressure.

But if you are exercising, your arteries are more likely to be pliable. They can more easily dilate (widen) so your blood pressure does not shoot way up to cause subsequent problems.

Through regular exercise and an active life, stress can have far fewer negative effects on your physical being. That, coupled with exercise's ability to improve sleep, can have profound positive effects on your mind, emotions, and spirit.

CHAPTER 7

EXERCISE AND OUR BRAIN

As we grow older, most everyone experiences changes in thinking ability and memory recall. It is pretty much considered a given and expected.

Fortunately, *physical activity can actually offset and prevent* much of the cognitive decline and memory loss that typically occurs over time with aging.

It can also help counter the more serious cognitive issues of Alzheimer's and Parkinson's, as well as depression.

Exercise Enhances Thinking

There are three mechanisms by which exercise helps cognitive function.

First is maintenance of cerebral blood flow. When you exercise, you are sending more oxygen-containing blood to the brain.

Second is the increase in *BDNF*, which stands for brain-derived neurotrophic factor. Elevated levels of BDNF help produce new neurons (nerve cells) in the brain, which leads to better function. In fact, not only do you acquire greater numbers of these healthy nerve cells, but communication between the nerve cells also improves as they send neurotransmitters between one another.

BDNF can be significantly increased by either of the following:

- Long-term aerobic exercise (thirty minutes, three times weekly for a year)
- Short-term vigorous exercise (such as soccer, tennis, or swimming for fifteen to thirty minutes, three times a week for at least three months)

The third benefit is that exercise enhances *brain volume* and *cognitive reserve*. Brain volume (mass) has been shown to increase when one is physically active. This limits the brain shrinking and atrophy that normally occurs as you age. This increases cognitive reserve (resistance to damage of the brain) and the number of healthy brain cells available, boosting your thinking processes.

Exercise Enhances Memory

Memory also improves with exercise. An area in the brain called the hippocampus deals primarily with memory. Starting at the age of forty, this hippocampus typically shrinks 1 to 2 percent per year, which can affect our recall ability. Again, exercise slows this decrease. In fact, physical activity *promotes* growth and so can retard future memory and possibly improve its present state.

Yet exercise does even more than help our thinking and recall abilities.

Alzheimer's Disease

Many have seen a parent or other loved one experience Alzheimer's heartbreaking effects, leading to early mortality. These people worry this condition may strike them some day as well.

They are justified in this concern. Alzheimer's is the sixth most common cause of death in the United States. The disease process starts with loss of short-term memory, and progresses until they no longer know family members or even who they are. This mental decline also negatively affects function in other organs, which eventually results in death.

It is of great concern to the aging population as the likelihood of an Alzheimer's diagnosis doubles every five years for someone over sixty-five years old.

While not everything is known about Alzheimer's, it has been determined that those suffering from this condition develop amyloid plaque in nerve cells in the memory portion of their brain. There are medications that can help diminish the symptoms *somewhat*, but at this point, there are no cures.

Alzheimer's is different from dementia, a more general term for serious memory loss and cognitive decline that interferes with daily living. Alzheimer's is actually the most common type of dementia as 60 to 80 percent of dementia patients develop Alzheimer's. One difference is people with dementia *that is not Alzheimer's* have not developed amyloid plaque, the hallmark of Alzheimer's.

Interestingly, some of the risk factors for Alzheimer's and dementia are very similar to those for heart disease.

Determining Who Will Get Alzheimer's

While presently impossible to predict who will get Alzheimer's, researchers have discovered certain risk factors common to Alzheimer's and coronary illness:

- Poor diet
- Overweight and obesity
- Hypertension
- Diabetes

From these overlaps, a guiding phrase has developed: What's good for the heart is good for the brain.

To help prevent Alzheimer's, people should be eating unsaturated fats, such as those in nuts, fish, and vegetable oils. A University of Chicago study led to the creation of the *MIND* diet. It is a combination of the Mediterranean diet and the DASH diet (the Americanized version of the Mediterranean diet), both of which are detailed in our chapter on Hypertension.

MIND is an acronym for

- Mediterranean and DASH diet
- Intervention
- Neural degenerative
- Delay

This MIND diet lowers the likelihood of developing Alzheimer's disease by 53 percent!

Not only that, if you exercise thirty minutes, three times a week, that can also lower chances for the onset of Alzheimer's disease.

Plus, exercise can slow the progression in patients *who already have Alzheimer's.*

How Exercise Helps Alzheimer's

As said earlier, exercise increases *BDNF* in the brain. It also combats Alzheimer's because it has a protective effect against the toxicity of amyloid plaque.

Interestingly, though *moving from moderate to vigorous exercise* will not make that much difference to cardiovascular health, *it provides more benefit faster* with Alzheimer's. That is because people with Alzheimer's will have low BDNF.

The bottom line is that Alzheimer's patients should exercise, and continue to exercise, for as long as possible. Caretakers should push their Alzheimer's patients to stay physically active.

Further Research Supports Being Active

A newer study of Alzheimer's was reported in the *Journal of Alzheimer's Disease* in June of 2017. They looked at people with high risk of developing Alzheimer's, those who had one gene variation linked to Alzheimer's or those who had one parent with the disease.

Neither group had yet developed cognitive dysfunction. The researchers looked deeper within these groups at those people who were doing light, moderate, or vigorous exercise.

They found that those who were doing light exercise (walking) were not getting any benefit.

Moderate exercise promoted healthy glucose metabolism in the brain, which means the overall brain activity is better (Alzheimer's patients have low glucose metabolism).

They then looked at those who did vigorous exercise. It benefited the hippocampus (memory), but not the other regions of the brain.

Their conclusion was that *moderate exercise provided a larger over-all cognitive benefit*, while *vigorous exercise gave a quick positive response to improving memory*.

Parkinson's Disease

Parkinson's is a disease where depletion of a neurotransmitter called *dopamine* in the brain results in communication issues between nerve cells. The result is patients experience resting tremors in hands, plus balance and muscle coordination problems such that they have slowed movement and difficulty walking, speaking, or performing simple tasks. They also exhibit a glum face without smiles or laughter.

It affects 1.5 million people in the United States, with seventy thousand new cases each year.

A December 2017 study in *JAMA Neurology* (*Journal of Medical Association Neurology*) followed patients who were diagnosed with Parkinson's but were not yet on medication.

Patients were divided into three groups:

- Those who did high-intensity exercise three times a week—meaning exercise that raises heart rate to 80 to 85 percent of your *predicted maximum* (220 minus your age)
- Moderate-intensity exercise three times a week—60 to 65 percent of predicted maximum heart rate
- No exercise at all

They found patients who did high-intensity exercise had symptoms that remained stable (the Parkinson's did not progress) or actually improved.

Those performing moderate-intensity exercise had symptoms worsen by 7.5 percent. Yet that was still a positive effect because those patients that *did not* exercise had symptoms worsen by 15 percent.

So moderate-intensity exercise helped slow down the progression of symptoms, while high-intensity kept patients stable and even offered improvement.

A significant finding.

Again, I remind readers that you *do not start off* by doing intense exercise. People that get heart attacks from exercise are primarily those that switch suddenly from a sedentary lifestyle to vigorous exercise. One should begin with light to moderate exercise and slowly advance to a higher intensity.

In addition to Alzheimer's, dementia, and Parkinson's, there is an even more common form of cognitive dysfunction we should discuss.

Depression

According to World Health Organization, depression is a leading cause of disability on a global level. In fact, it is more frequently seen in industrial countries.

So how do doctors diagnose depression?

There are two major and seven minor criteria. You need to have at least one of the major criteria and at least four of the minor criteria to be given a diagnosis of *clinical depression.*

The major criteria are as follows:

+ A constantly depressed mood
+ Loss of interest in everyday activities once enjoyed and engaged in

The seven minor criteria are as follows:

+ Change of appetite
+ Sleep problems
+ Fatigue
+ Feeling of hopelessness
+ Difficulty in thinking
+ Agitation
+ Thoughts of suicide

So how is depression typically treated?

A common treatment is medication. But there is the problem of side effects. There are even combination medications, which have even more side effects. These can include headaches, nausea, dizziness, sexual dysfunction, sleep problems, and others.

Psychologists can also treat depression with cognitive behavioral therapy. This helps patients develop problem-solving skills.

But there is another remedy to be considered.

Exercise.

A large-scale study in the January 2018 issue of the *American Journal of Psychiatry* followed 32,908 patients for eleven years. They looked at what percentage of these people developed anxiety or depression during that time and what role exercise could play.

The study found that one hour per week of *any* intensity exercise prevented the incidence of depression. The conclusion is that it does not take that much exercise to lower the likelihood of developing this disorder. The exercise can be light, moderate, or vigorous.

Irony of Using Our Brain and Exercise

It is noteworthy to recognize that the majority of people with sedentary jobs are primarily using their minds for work. That is how they earn a living, how they may feel valued in the world. Yet what are they doing to maintain or improve their ability to think or their memory? Coffee? Energy drinks? Staring at a TV screen at night to relax?

Also available to them is regular exercise and/or sports that can yield not only a wide range of benefits as described elsewhere in this book, exercise can improve the very thing they are relying upon for their livelihood and self-worth!

That can give them that competitive edge.

Of course, you do not need to be at a desk job to gain these benefits. As we have read, improving and extending our lifelong ability to think and recall, avoiding brain-related ailments and the hidden epidemic of depression, is a wonderful gift that no person in their right mind would want to ignore.

So get moving!

CHAPTER 8

EXERCISE AND CANCER

One of the most frightening words that people can hear is *cancer*.

It brings up thoughts of a devastating, often fatal disease that seems to strike without warning. There are between 1.5 and 1.7 million new diagnoses of cancer every year in the United States. For many individuals, it is the one illness that worries them most, even though more lives are lost to heart disease every year than to cancers.

Cancer worries may surpass those of heart disease because people think there are steps they can take to reduce the likelihood of getting heart disease and recovering from it. Yet there *are* ways to help prevent cancers and help recovery too.

One of those ways is, you guessed it—exercise.

The good news is there are, again, profound benefits to exercise. Exercise is helpful for preventing cancer, for people being treated for cancer, and for those people whose cancer has gone into remission.

Benign and Malignant Tumors

To begin, let us understand the difference between benign and malignant tumors. The distinction is simple: If you have abnormal cells growing that stay local (within an organ, for instance), it is called benign. It only affects the local area, and in most cases, if that diseased portion is removed (usually surgically), the patient should recover well.

71

Abnormal cells termed malignant are those that spread though the blood or lymphatic system to other organs. These are then called cancer. The cells continue replicating with their mutated DNA. These cells are the most dangerous and capable of killing people as they damage organs in many areas of the body.

Contributors to Cancer

What makes cancers form in the first place?

While theories vary, the factors that determine formation are most commonly thought to be twofold: the environment (originating from outside the body) and a genetic predisposition toward the disease (sourcing from the body's inherent makeup). If issues exist with both of these, the probability is greater that a person can end up with cancer.

Among environmental causes, first and foremost is smoking as 25 to 30 percent of all cancer deaths are attributed to this activity. It primarily manifests as lung cancer, but smoking can contribute to cancers in other organs as well.

Perhaps surprising to many people is that obesity and a sedentary lifestyle can together contribute to 25 percent of cancers, especially breast and colon cancers. So there is immediately strong evidence that exercise can prevent cancers because if you are not obese and you are physically active, your chances of getting breast or colon cancer diminish greatly.

Infections of some viruses and bacteria contribute to 15 to 20 percent of cancers. For example, certain strains of the human papillomavirus (HPV) can cause cervical cancers in women, while chronic *Helicobacter pylori* infections in the stomach wall can result in gastric carcinoma.

Radiation from medical x-rays, CAT (CT) scans, fluoroscopy, etc.—as well as UV radiation from the sun—can damage cells, causing 10 percent of cancers.

Exposure to toxic chemicals and poor air quality have also been linked to cancers.

While stress rightfully gets attention as a potential cause, stress alone accounts for less than 10 percent of incidents of cancer. But it *can contribute* to development of cancers from other causes.

While all these environmental sources are justifiably of concern, it should be noted that the causes (smoking and obesity and sedentary lifestyle) of 50 percent of cancers are *preventable.*

Hormones

Another contributing factor to certain cancers is hormones, primarily estrogen, which has been linked to breast, uterine, and ovarian cancers.

Immune System Protection

The reality is that our bodies are constantly exposed to things, which, if left unchecked (such as infections, cell mutations, etc.), can turn into cancer. One of the primary means by which this is avoided is with an effective immune system. Time and again our immune system neutralizes these threats, fighting off germs and infections. In addition, as the body keeps replicating cells, sometimes errors may occur, and there is rapid cell death. A healthy immune system clears out these cells before they become malignant.

If one has a weakened immune system due to infections or other causes, then the system will be less able to clear out these replicating error cells and prevent them from turning into cancer.

Oncogenes

Each of our body's cells has proto-oncogenes. These act on a cellular level to promote normal and healthy cell growth. But radiation or viruses can affect proto-oncogenes and turn them into oncogenes. The oncogenes, unfortunately, can cause uncontrolled growth that replicate cells that may not be healthy.

Prevention: Exercise

Obviously, some ways in which we can prevent cancers is to limit our exposure to environmental contributors. Refraining from smoking has already been cited. The array of toxic chemicals that we may be exposed to on a daily basis are extensive (including many household cleansers, pesticides in food, etc.), yet we often have the option for healthier choices. But other potential causes are not so easily eluded. We have no choice but to breathe the air around us (unless we move to healthier environs).

But there is one thing that should *not* be avoided, something that can profoundly assist the avoidance of developing cancers.

Again, exercise.

Studies Provide the Proof

A review of forty-eight different studies, encompassing 40,000 patients, showed that exercise reduces risks of colon cancer by a range of 10 to 70 percent. It is believed the reason is that exercise makes the bowels move better and thus reduce the bowel transit time, so there is less opportunity for the waste byproducts of food to spend time in the colon and expose the body to toxins.

There have also been forty-one other studies, comprising 108,000 patients, documenting that exercise reduces incidence of breast cancer by 30 percent.

Additionally, research has shown that exercise reduces endometrial cancer (the inner lining of the uterus) by 10 to 80 percent.

Never Too Late to Start but Perhaps Best to Start Early

Negating the false notion of people not previously on an exercise regimen who may think it is too late for them—the most preventive benefits have been shown to be for patients who went from a sedentary lifestyle of low fitness—to an active routine encompassing moderate fitness. On the other hand, there does not appear to be that much benefit to increasing from moderate fitness to high level fitness.

But this does not mean one should wait until they are older (or worse, until they have cancer) to become physically active.

There are theories that people active in sports starting when they are young may help prevent certain cancers from occurring later during middle age or later in life. That is because some cancers take many years to develop and must initiate when one is young for the cancer to have enough time to develop within a person's lifetime.

What Amount Is the Right Amount?

While some studies simply have determined significant benefit to exercise in regard to cancer, other studies have looked at *how much activity* is actually needed.

They calculate this by determining the number of calories that must be burned up each week through exercise. Most studies found that expending one thousand calories per week (equaling about four hours total of moderate activity or three hours total of vigorous activity) can significantly protect against colon, breast, and lung cancer.

Note: one should not conclude that exercise will not *also* protect against other types of cancers beyond the ones mentioned. It is simply that the most extensive studies so far have focused on these specific diseases.

Exercise Is Great Prevention Except When It Is Too Much

If you are sedentary, your immune system is typically not functioning well. Yet if you exercise moderately or vigorously, your immune system becomes stronger and more viable.

However, those people that go *beyond* moderate and vigorous to more excessive and exhaustive regimens such as training for and participating in marathons, triathlons, and CrossFit programs actually *weaken* their immune system. They cause it to become less effective than even those of sedentary people.

As you will see me say many times in this book and have undoubtedly heard from others, *moderation is key.*

People participating in such excessive exercise are *pushing beyond* what their bodies are designed to do.

This self-induced damage will weaken more than just the immune system. It can also cause or accelerate heart disease (detailed in the chapter on endurance sports). If one pushes themselves into exhaustive exercise, there is actually cardiac cell death. You are producing harm. Another common and more immediate effect of this level of activity is upper respiratory tract infections.

Strategy to Prevent Breast Cancer: Start Exercise Early

Breast cancer is of major concern to women. Yet there is another means by which one can help prevent its occurrence. It is connected to the woman's reproductive life cycle and hormones.

Ovulation releases large amounts of estrogen and progesterone. However, too much estrogen can fuel breast cancer growth. The less time a woman is ovulating, the lower the risk of cancer. Ovulation is interrupted during pregnancy. A woman who does not bear children (or go through pregnancy) may have a higher chance for breast cancer. Of course, ovulation is permanently over when the woman goes through menopause. In fact, if a woman goes through menopause before the age of forty-five, her risk of cancer is much lower than if she enters menopause after the age of fifty-five.

It should be noted, however, that women in postmenopause who are overweight are instead *more prone* to breast cancer as they have more fat. Estrogen stores in fat cells.

At the other end of this time spectrum, studies have shown that if you delay when a young woman has her first period, there is less chance she will develop breast cancer in the future. When the onset of periods (also called *menarche*) begins before the age of twelve, there is much higher risk of breast cancer than if it begins at age thirteen or later.

And here is the reason why I bring this up: Menarche can be postponed if girls are actively exercising.

When menarche is delayed, ovulation and its release of estrogen and progesterone is delayed as well. In fact, for every year it is postponed, the cancer risk reduces by 5 to 15 percent.

Unfortunately, we are seeing girls starting periods at younger and younger ages. This may relate to younger people being less active (spending more time on computers and smartphones playing video games and other activities), eating a poorer diet, and the occurrence of more childhood obesity.

Exercise while Having Cancer

If someone has been diagnosed with cancer, they should not assume it is too late for them to start exercising.

On the contrary.

Studies have shown that exercise *can counter* the promotion of cancer cell replication and *slows down* the cancer's development. If you are diagnosed with cancer, even before you start chemo or other treatment, begin routine exercise. Aside from reducing cell replication, it also decreases anxiety and helps empower your immune system.

Exercise should continue as you undergo chemotherapy as well. Now going through chemotherapy is very challenging. It puts great strain on the body and on a person's mental state. Yet it has been shown that even when one is receiving chemotherapy, results are better if they exercise. A person's anxiety reduces, there is less stress, and they sleep better—all of which helps the immune system fight the cancer.

Strategize the Exercise

So how best to exercise when chemo is making someone weak and tired? Aside from choosing the right level of exercise for an individual's physical state at the time, they must choose when to do them. As chemo's greatest negative side effects occur a few days after treatment and is when the person feels most tired and sick, that is obviously a time to take a break from exercise. But during other times, continue to be active.

Cancer Patients Who Should Not Exercise

While I champion exercise for preventing cancers and for those who have cancer, there are certain people with cancer who *should not* be exercising. These would include individuals who have the following:

- Hemoglobin levels of less than 10 (anemic)
- Extremely low white blood cell counts below 3,000
- Low platelet counts (platelets help blood coagulation) below 50,000
- Fevers above 100.4 Fahrenheit (38 degrees centigrade)
- Shortness of breath at rest (sitting or lying down)
- Bone pain (that could mean the cancer has spread to bones, which could fracture from exercise)
- An unsteady gait (unstable walking, affected by nerves; we do not want to risk them falling and breaking something)

Some of these conditions can be side effects of chemotherapy. Patients should wait until the above symptoms have subsided before resuming exercise.

Exercise for Patients in Remission after Treatment

Studies have shown that moderate exercise of 150 minutes per week can decrease recurrence of breast cancer by 50 percent.

Alternatively, research indicates people need double that amount of moderate exercise—three hundred minutes per week—to reduce colon cancer recurrence.

While there have not been conclusive studies showing the amounts of moderate exercise needed to help prevent recurrence of other cancers, physical activity is still likely to help avert recurrence of other cancers as well.

Powerful Tool for Health

As you are beginning to see, exercise helps counter a wide scope of medical conditions, including many that we are not even addressing.

As the addition of this chapter attests, being physically active helps to offset the *two illnesses most responsible for deaths* in the United States: cardiovascular disease and cancer. That alone should motivate people to seek out opportunities to adopt an active lifestyle.

ATHLETES ARE NOT EXEMPT

Understanding Health Risks

CHAPTER 9

FEAR OF EXERCISE

Playing It Safe So You Can Play

As I have said, given the extraordinary value of physical activity, one might expect pretty much everyone would engage in some form of exercise program.

But many do not.

We have heard all the usual reasons: I'm too tired… There's not enough time… Don't know what kinds of exercises to do… There are too many new things to watch on TV.

While I called these reasons, they are actually excuses. Ones mostly born out if inertia or ignorance.

Yet some people refrain for a very valid reason: fear.

They know or suspect they have health issues, they have been sedentary, and they are worried about harming themselves. *They are afraid to start exercising.* The truth is, there is a potential for heart attacks, strokes, or sudden death if patients do not understand how to exercise properly for their condition.

One of the primary purposes of this book is to share the types and levels of exercise that are most appropriate for you and how to proceed with them in a safe and effective manner.

I have seen exercise create stunning turnarounds in patient health, changing lives for the better. I have also seen disasters, most often when I am called into a case with someone who had not been my

83

patient but has now *become* my patient after they experience a cardiac event.

An event I know could have been prevented.

At Most Risk

Let us start by recognizing that one of the highest-risk groups are the so-called weekend warriors, individuals sedentary throughout the week who then play in a vigorous weekend game of softball, soccer, basketball, or other strenuous activity. It may be a sport in which they participated when they were young and see no reason not to do so again.

But now, there may be reasons.

In fact, such perils are not confined only to those wishing to participate in a sport or even a defined exercise regimen. I have seen a retired farmer who had been sedentary buy a house with land and start farming again. Even though he had performed that kind of work most of his life, he was now doing more than his body could handle. He was found in the field, deceased. I know this scenario because of farms near my area in the Central Valley.

But it does not have to be this way.

Exercise Is Just One Component of Good Health

Though I discuss the advantages of exercise and how to safely do it, exercise should not be seen as the sole contributor to a long, healthy life.

While exercise can certainly blunt and even reverse the effects of aging, the right diet is also needed. Plus, if someone has a strong family history of heart disease, they should visit a cardiologist for testing before embarking on a new exercise program (or frankly, even if they are already exercising). If someone has hypertension, it must be treated. Diabetes must be treated. Exercise may reduce health risks but not necessarily eliminate them. Not all by itself.

We need to be smart and realistic about participating in an exercise program.

Family History of Heart Disease?

Let us start with this question: What defines family history?

Anyone having a parent or sibling or uncle or aunt that has had a heart attack or stroke, or that died suddenly because of a heart condition, before the age of fifty-five for a man or sixty-five for a woman, is considered someone with a positive family history for heart disease. A person with such a history, even if they are already athletes and perform marathons and are eating well, should routinely see a cardiologist to test if they are developing blockages or other underlying conditions.

If those issues do exist, it is far better to deal with it before it causes a medical crisis. Not wanting to know (as some people are inclined) does not make those conditions go away. Actually, the opposite. It allows them to surprisingly, and unpleasantly, affect your life. Or end it.

When a Cardiologist Is Needed Rather Than Your GP

If you simply have hypertension and only want to walk for exercise, having your medical general practitioner monitor you is fine.

But if you want to participate in any vigorous activity, such as running, soccer, basketball, or swimming, I recommend being checked by a cardiologist. Best would be someone competent in sports cardiology.

Admittedly, there is not an abundance of sports cardiologists, those doctors with an added specialty focusing on athletes or patients interested in starting an exercise program. I am probably the only one in Northern California, along with a few at Stanford. I know this as I am on the Sports Cardiology Council for the United States. But such physicians are out there, often at academic centers where sports cardiology is all that they do.

There are also those like me who do everything that a cardiologist normally would do, focusing on patients of all ages as well as those participating at all levels of physical activity. While you may not live near a doctor who has this added specialty, you certainly want a cardiologist who is knowledgeable about this subject, including knowledge of the appropriate exercise regimens for different individuals at different levels of fitness.

Exercise Prescriptions

One might look at exercising as they might driving a car. Driving can enhance our life immeasurably. In fact, most adults in the United States have a driver's license. But you need to *learn* to drive, or you risk dramatic negative consequences.

You also need to learn about proper exercise.

That means the proper exercise *for you.* You should have an exercise prescription specifically designed for you. The most specific ones would likely come from a sports cardiologist or perhaps an exercise physiologist or some other specialist in sport medicine with an understanding of how to prescribe exercises for different types of patients. In general, I suggest that an individual with a family history of heart disease or other risk factors who is seeking to undertake an exercise program should see their general practitioner for a referral to a sports cardiologist or sports medicine specialist.

This book will offer general guidelines to aid in understanding what kinds of exercises may be appropriate for you (and why) and who in particular needs to see a sports cardiologist before starting on a physically active program.

For You and Those around You

My goal is that readers of this book gain insight and understanding not only about your own fitness situation but also that of your loved ones. Your children may someday be involved in sports programs or have health issues. At the other end of the spectrum, this information is also critical if you have aging parents or other older relatives and friends.

If you are already an athlete, then you, too, want a greater understanding so you can perform the best that you can safely.

Athletes Are Not Exempt

Negative cardiac or other medical events can potentially occur to anyone who is physically active. This *includes* even professional athletes, those who are thought of as the epitome of healthy individuals. As active as they are, they still have human bodies, and those bodies can have issues that must be addressed.

Many of us have heard of well-known athletes who experienced heart attacks or sudden death. The tragic story of Hank Gathers is such an example: a twenty-three-year-old American college basketball player who collapsed during a game in 1990 and died.

In the United States, the most common cause of sudden death in athletes is *hypertrophic cardiomyopathy*. People need a genetic disposition toward this disease in order to have it. Curiously, such a person is usually normal during childhood. The heart functions well. But as they hit adolescence or young adulthood, the genetics kick in, and part of their heart muscle becomes thickened (hypertrophied).

This can lead to symptoms and possibly syncope (passing out). That is because this thickened region occurs at the outflow tract where the heart's left ventricle pumps blood to the rest of the body. This obstructs the blood flow, especially during exercise, when not enough blood pumps from the heart to vital organs. The brain, for example, may not receive sufficient oxygen from the blood, and the person can pass out. They may recover and get up again after the heart restabilizes. But they will continue to experience chest pains, shortness of breath, etc.

This is what happened to Hank Gathers. He passed out twice, was examined, and found to have arrhythmias during exercise. So he was given beta-blockers medication in order to stabilize this condition. But he *should* have been stopped from playing entirely. Because even with the beta-blockers, you can develop arrhythmias (abnormal heart rhythm, meaning it does not beat properly) because you have *two things* going on with hypertrophic cardiomyopathy: the thickened muscle, plus the way that these muscles developed when he was born.

It is like constructing a building. If you have not laid the bricks in the right places, the building is unstable. In a similar way, the muscles of the heart in people like Hank Gathers were not formed correctly. A disarray of muscle cells causes arrhythmias. When that becomes a form of arrhythmia called *ventricular tachycardia*, the electrical impulses that stimulate the heart muscle to contract do so improperly. In essence, the pump is ineffective, and you can pass out.

Plus, ventricular tachycardia can lead to *ventricular fibrillation* (V-fib), an even more serious condition where the heart essentially just shivers slightly and does not really contract at all. When this happens, unless you have access to a defibrillator and apply it immediately to shock the heart and restore the electrical rhythm, these people usually die. This is why it is so important to have AEDs (automated external defibrillators) accessible at sporting events so they can be quickly applied. That is the reason I was so heavily involved in getting AEDs into sports programs at the local high schools in my area. They save lives.

That is probably what happened to Hank Gathers when he played again in his last game. As I said, doctors had put him on beta-blockers, and he continued competing, thinking he was fine to play. But Hank did not like the side effects of beta-blockers as they make you tired, so there is some uncertainty whether he took his medication on the day of his last game. Most likely, he had a malignant arrhythmia (serious and life-threatening), and they were unable to revive him.

That incident pushed the medical field to better evaluate college and professional athletes with EKGs and with a different health questionnaire than we use for the general public. At the same time, this made it more important to understand that when someone has symptoms, it is imperative to work with them to come up with guidelines as to when they may perform different activities at different levels, based upon their diagnosis.

Further exacerbating the situation is that some athletes with this condition are consuming performance-enhancing drugs, such as energy drinks, that can stimulate the heart inappropriately.

Your Voyage to Healthy Exercise

While there are indeed conditions and circumstances that can make exercise risky for certain individuals at any level of fitness, the intent of this book is to make you smarter about exercise so you will have the confidence to do it properly without fear of causing yourself harm. You can perform better, more safely, and enjoy the improved quality of living that results from a lifelong commitment to physical activity.

Remember this: You do not have to be in great shape to start exercising. Most people coming to exercise are not. What you do need is new awareness and perhaps a doctor who can guide your journey.

CHAPTER 10

NO ONE IS IMMUNE

Athletes Get Symptoms Too

Since physical activity and exercise puts extra demands on our heart and coronary system, readers need to recognize various symptoms that might occur and why. This way you will know to pay attention and when to consult a physician.

This is true for everyone, including top athletes.

In fact, if you are active, you are more prone to discover you have a blockage earlier than someone who is not active. Why?

The reason is supply and demand. During active exercise, the demand on your heart goes up. If you have a blockage, your heart cannot supply enough oxygenated blood through your body. You have symptoms. Someone sedentary who never really exerts themselves will not know if they have blockages because they do not raise the demand enough on the heart.

But it is a plus for people who exercise to find out and get it treated sooner, before it becomes a more severe issue that causes a massive heart attack. So now the benefit to exercising is *at least twofold*: Not only does exercise increase your likelihood for better health and life, exercising can also increase the likelihood of discovering an issue earlier while it is easier to correct.

Starting with an Exam

I often have professional athletes referred to my practice for a preparticipation exam before they begin vigorous exercise. I have contracts with several professional teams, including the Sacramento Republic FC soccer team, whose athletes come to me for clearance.

But most of those coming to my office are high school and college athletes, along with the general populace, who do not come in for the precise cardiovascular exam that we conduct for our professional athletes. The majority of these patients are seeing me because of a symptom. These are most often passing out (syncope), heart racing (palpitations), chest pains, or shortness of breath beyond what is expected from the activity.

We start the exam by getting a medical history on the patient, including history of any cardiovascular disease in their family. This would include if anyone in their immediate family, plus uncles or aunts, ever had sudden cardiac death (also called cardiac arrest). That would certainly raise a red flag, especially in regard to those embarking on athletics.

With athletes—who always want to perform better than others—I also inquire if they are taking any kind of enhancing agents. Examples can include anabolic steroids, which can elevate blood pressure. Or erythropoietin, a substance normally released by the kidneys to stimulate the bone marrow to make more red blood cells (and thus deliver more performance-enhancing oxygen). Erythropoietin poses risks as well as too many red blood cells traveling through tiny vessels can cause blockages that lead to heart attacks. (A later chapter on misuse of drugs goes into further detail.)

But let me now address some of the most common symptoms that bring those participating in athletics to my office.

Syncope

Though perhaps not well-known to the general public, it is not uncommon for athletes to occasionally pass out. That might sound like a serious condition, but passing out can be benign (little detrimental effect) or what we call malignant (threatening to life). In either case, there is concern that an athlete could injure themselves from a fall while passing out.

In its most basic form, syncope is where the heart does not pump enough oxygen-containing blood to the brain. You pass out due to a temporary shortage of oxygen in the brain, after which sufficient blood flow resumes, and you stand up again.

There is also a term called *presyncope*, which means light-headedness. You *feel like you might* pass out, but you do not. Both need to be examined.

Looking Deeper

When we consider syncope in athletes, we first place it in one of three categories. Does the passing out occur *after exercise, during exercise,* or *before exercise?*

Passing out *before* exercise is most likely related to the athlete being anxious.

Yet passing out *during exercise* is our biggest red flag and potentially highly dangerous. We need to discover what caused it.

Passing Out After Exercise

Let me first explain passing out *after exercise* since it is the most common of the three scenarios. Fortunately, it has a benign diagnosis.

This is what happens: when exercising, your total peripheral resistance reduces. That is, your arteries dilate (widen) to allow more needed blood flow to your various body parts. But this also causes the blood pressure to drop, and this could cause you to pass out if not enough blood reaches your brain. Fortunately, the body can counterbalance this when you move your legs. The contracting leg muscles squeeze the blood vessels in your legs, which then pump more blood back to your heart (called the *venous return*).

So even though your arteries carrying blood from the heart to the body are dilated, the veins in your legs are sending more blood back to the heart, increasing the amount of blood in the heart. This can offset the lower pressure in the dilated arteries.

While you are running, you are not going to pass out. *But once you suddenly stop*, there is no more leg movement. Your arteries are still dilated, but the venous return (sending blood back to the heart) abruptly reduces. The lowered artery blood pressures are not counteracted, and the person can lose consciousness.

Interestingly, this phenomenon tends to occur more frequently in women than men, though it is not known why.

So how do we prevent this from happening? First off, you should always do a cool down after you exercise. For example, if having a run, then jog or walk.

Do not just suddenly stop.

Second, if this light-headedness or passing out seems to be a repeated pattern for you, drink more fluids. By consuming extra fluids before and during exercise, the volume of fluid in your blood stream is greater, which can offset the issue even when your venous return is lower. Some might recommend taking fluids with more sodium in it, but I would not recommend that in general. This might be fine for young athletes, but not for those who are older.

Third, you could wear compressive stockings (socks) to squeeze the legs. This squeezes the veins as well, which yields the same effect as if your muscles are squeezing them.

What I have described here as a benign condition is simply due to a normal reaction of the body. That does not mean one has any kind of disease.

However, if you pass out *during* exercise, that is when we really delve deeper.

Passing Out during Exercise

If passing out during exercise is caused by blood pressure suddenly dropping, there most likely is some issue with the heart.

If blood pressure drops *slowly*, it may be related to seizures. In some cases, you may experience symptoms indicating that passing out is imminent (something doctors call prodrome). Most heart-related syncope is sudden: you are awake, and then you are out. However, if it is neurological, you get a quick warning such as tunnel vision or light-headedness or dizziness, and then you pass out. Because of this warning, these noncardiac causes of syncope result in less injuries than cardiac-caused syncope, since you have time to prepare before you fall (and pass out).

Other conditions can be involved if a young athlete passes out while exercising:

- Ventricular tachycardia
- Long QT syndrome (a genetic disease that relates to how fast the heart relaxes after contraction)
- Brugada syndrome
- Supraventricular tachycardia (SVC)
- Hypertrophic cardiomyopathy
- Arrhythmogenic right ventricular cardiomyopathy (ARVC)
- Myocarditis (inflammation of the heart)
- Coronary anomaly

Other Heart Conditions in Athletes

One might expect that athletes, who tend to have physical fitness that is superior to the average person's, would be more immune to heart issues. While it is true that exercise bestows considerable health advantages, athletes are still susceptible to cardiac disorders.

In fact, since athletes push themselves to perform at the highest levels, demanding more of their bodies, symptoms of underlying ailments can appear earlier than they might otherwise and with greater intensity.

Let us address other symptoms of heart problems that can commonly affect athletes. These will include the following:

- Palpitations
- Chest pains
- Extreme fatigue or performance decline

Palpitations

Palpitations are feelings of pounding and/or very rapid heartbeats. It is very uncomfortable and can occur suddenly while exercising.

So how serious is this?

That depends. It is critical to recognize the timing of when the palpitations occur in relation to exertion: does it happen before, during, or after exercise?

There is less concern if felt *before exercise*.

But if palpitations occur *while you are exercising*, that can be dangerous if either of these apply:

- There are symptoms of *presyncope* (light-headed feeling like you will pass out, but do not) or actual syncope (you pass out).
- The patient has had a family member—parent, grandparent, siblings, aunt/uncle—who had sudden cardiac death. This may alert us that syncope is probably secondary to some genetic predisposition (tendency) to arrhythmias such as long QT syndrome or hypertrophic cardiomyopathy.

Either of these two scenarios could be severe and life-threatening and must be explored further. A starting point is always to ask the athlete if they are using drugs, including stimulants such as caffeine or anything related to ephedrine. Any use of stimulants can cause or worsen palpitations.

PVCs and PACs

Palpitations felt *after exercise* could be PVCs (*premature ventricular complex*) or PACs (*premature atrial complex*).

If the athlete *did not feel* as if they might pass out from this, or if a doctor confirms there is no structural heart disease (such as valve or heart muscle problems or congenital issues), *and the palpitations go away when exercising*, then this is not of concern. That is because arrhythmia that only occur occasionally and are not related to disease (not due to blockages or a weakened heart) typically get better with exercise. The arrhythmia result from stress, and routine exercise relieves stress.

Atrial Flutter

However, if our workup includes the athlete wearing a *Holter monitor* (portable electrocardiogram device that records heart electrical activity over twenty-four hours), and there are more than 2,000 irregular heartbeats (PACs) in a twenty-four-hour period, this is serious, and we look deeper for the reason, as it can mean you are inclined toward atrial fibrillation, a much more dangerous issue. (Note: While 2,000 irregular heartbeats might sound unfathomably high to some readers, keep in mind that a person with a typical heart rate of 70 beats per minute has 100,800 total beats in a normal twenty-four-hour period.) Also, if you have over 20,000 PVCs in twenty-four hours, then you are at risk of developing cardiomyopathy.

We search for what may cause the patient to develop such symptoms, especially as they may lead to "exercise intolerance" (reduced capacity to perform at the athlete's normal ability or duration). One possibility is *atrial flutter*. This is a common arrhythmia that starts in a portion of the atrium, resulting in *regular but rapid* contractions, ultimately causing the heart to beat around 150 beats per minute or higher.

Keep in mind this is different than AFib (atrial fibrillation), an arrhythmia that also starts in the atrium but produces irregular and chaotic beats. (AFib is actually more common in competitive athletes than in the general public.)

V-tach

If the Holter monitor reveals that the athlete has *ventricular tachycardia* (V-tach), a rapid heartbeat over 100 beats per minute that starts in the ventricle, we have a dangerous situation. Some athletes with this arrhythmia may handle up to 150 beats per minute for a short period, but once the heart rate surpasses 150, it could cause a drop in blood pressure and passing out. The heart cannot pump enough blood, so the person can pass out. If this also causes the heart to not receive enough oxygen (due to insufficient blood flow to the heart muscle itself), the heart can go into total *ventricular fibrillation* and stop. That is how people die. While this can occur at any level of exercise, chances are increased with vigorous exercise.

A person with ventricular tachycardia needs a full workup, which can include an echocardiogram and a cardiac MRI, to determine if the patient has structural heart disease.

Additional Testing

Patients who have *arrhythmias with exercise* should also have blood tests to check thyroid function and iron levels. Excess iron can be a cause. It is possible the patient has hemochromatosis disease (usually an inherited condition) that causes excessive iron deposits in the body, including in the heart muscle. Anemia (a deficiency of healthy red blood cells to transport sufficient oxygen to body tissues) can also be a cause of palpitations. Electrolytes should also be checked. An echocardiogram should be performed.

Depending on what is found, we might treat the condition conservatively: instruct the patient to cut down on caffeine, energy drinks, not to binge drink, along with other possible habitual changes. We may treat with medications. These issues are reversible.

Lastly, if the arrhythmias can be treated, a *cardiac electrophysiologist* (a subspecialty of cardiology, also called an EP doctor) can use an electrical current to burn and eliminate the faulty electrical pathway or the area of the heart causing the arrhythmias. This is called ablation.

Chest Pain

"No pain, no gain" is not a slogan to apply when it comes to the heart. Pain is a warning signal that must be given attention. Something serious may be, or is about to be, occurring. You do not "tough it through" with the heart.

Particularly with chest pain.

Chest pains are not uncommon. Patients, from grade school through college and beyond, as well as professional athletes, come to my office with chest pains. Even while coaching my youth soccer teams, I have had players experience chest pain.

Though an often-seen symptom, it becomes extremely important for athletes *over thirty-five years old*. Then you must start thinking about coronary artery disease, which is what most frequently kills people.

Fortunately, cardiologists are well-equipped to determine the causes behind chest pain, when to advise a competitive player to suspend participation, and how to treat it.

Causes of Chest Pain

When discussing the causes of chest pain, it helps to divide them into four different categories:

- Coronary artery disorders
- Myocardial (heart muscle) causes
- Cardiac causes
- Noncardiac causes

Coronary Artery Disorders Causes of Chest Pain

For people over thirty-five, we especially want to look at the possibility of blockages in arteries. Those can be from the following:

- *Atherosclerosis*—one of the most common conditions, where plaque builds up on the inner lining of arteries. If this creates a thick blockage that inhibits sufficient blood flow during the high requirements of exercise, you may have chest pains (a heart attack is also possible). If you stop the exercise, the pain goes away. But if the next day you do the same exercise at the same level and get the same chest pain, this is indicative of a tight blockage. Typical symptoms can include chest pain with a feeling of pressure radiating to the neck or arm. You might also feel nausea.

+ *Anomalous coronary artery* (coronary artery anomalies)— the symptoms are very sporadic but usually manifest with very high-intensity exercise. The condition is due to a malformation in the heart that developed in the womb. The first arteries, which normally come out of a specific portion of the aorta to feed the heart, emerged instead from a *different* part of the aorta. This incorrect placement causes them to be *squeezed* as the heart pumps hard during intense exercise. That squeezing causes less blood flow to the heart (a similar effect as a blocked coronary artery). That means less oxygen and nutrients reach the heart muscle. It can produce arrhythmias that make the person pass out or even die.

+ *Coronary artery dissection*—the artery's inner lining separates from the rest of the artery wall and partially (or completely) blocks blood flow to the heart. The result is acute pain that *continues after* you stop exercising.

+ *Coronary artery vasospasm*—a tightening of the muscles in the artery wall, which then constricts blood flow to the heart. This spasm is not usually associated with exercise itself but is more likely felt due to emotional stress or cold weather.

Myocardial (Heart Muscle) Causes of Chest Pain

For patients *under* thirty-five years old, the most common causes of chest pain are *hypertrophic cardiomyopathy* and *coronary artery anomalies*:

+ *Hypertrophic cardiomyopathy* (HCM)—a genetic disorder that causes a malfunction in the heart muscle's formation such that it gets very thick. But this does not typically manifest itself until adolescence. When the heart muscle needs more oxygen during exercise, the heart is so thick that it cannot get enough to meet the demand. This is the most common cause of sudden cardiac death in young athletes in the United States.

+ *Myocarditis*—inflammation of the heart muscle cells. Or *Pericarditis*, inflammation of the two thin layers of tissue (pericardium) surrounding the heart muscle. Each of these can be caused by a virus, chemotherapy, or sometimes nutritional deficiencies. Myocarditis can cause chest pains, shortness of breath, or palpitations. Pericarditis can interfere with heart function and cause *sharp* chest pains that are positional (they intensify when you move, such as if you bend over or lay on your back or side). They feel different from a heart attack, which is accompanied by *pressure and tightness* in the chest.

Cardiac Causes of Chest Pain

These include the following:

+ *Myocardial* (heart muscle) *disorders*
+ *Aortic dissection*—a tear in the inner layer of the aorta, the large blood vessel branching off from the heart.
+ *Demand ischemia* (*ischemia* means a heart receives insufficient oxygen)—can result from hypertrophic cardiomyopathy, where the heart muscle is so thick that it cannot get enough oxygen.
+ *Valve disease*—which becomes apparent during the higher oxygen demands of exercise, when the impaired valve inhibits sufficient blood flow and nutrients going to the heart.

Non-Cardiac Causes of Chest Pain

Note that you will not immediately die from noncardiac sources:

+ *Asthma*—can create tightness in the chest, though is usually accompanied by wheezing or lung symptoms.

- *Pneumothorax*—is usually due to part of the lung spontaneously collapsing, yielding sharp chest pains when taking deep breaths, and is accompanied by shortness of breath. Tends to occur in very tall people.
- *Pneumonia*—though is usually accompanied with cough and fever.
- *Gastrointestinal symptoms*—such as acid reflux. Usually the pain is more burning and accompanied with belching and nausea.
- *Pulmonary embolism*—occurs when blood clots in a leg travel to the lungs. Suddenly there is acute chest pain while breathing, shortness of breath, and you may cough up blood. With such symptoms, the doctor asks a series of questions: Is there is a history of clotting in the family? Do you smoke? Are you using oral contraceptives? Have you been sitting without getting up for four to six hours (as can happen while traveling)? This lack of movement as a cause can be especially probable if you are obese. Though noncardiac, it should be noted that pulmonary embolism *can* be lethal.
- *Muscular skeletal issues*—most commonly seen in athletes, it could be a rib fracture or costochondritis (inflammatory joint pain where the cartilage attaches to ribs). The pain is very localized, such that placing your finger on an afflicted area will reveal it as the source of the discomfort. This can occur after exercise such as lifting weights, as happened to me. I had been weight training and a week later felt the pain while playing soccer.

Red Flag

While some of these aforementioned conditions are more serious than others, an overall red flag for chest pain occurs if it is accompanied with passing out or a feeling of almost passing out. This means the heart muscle is so stunned from not receiving enough oxygen that it is pumping poorly and the person gets light-headed since the heart is not sending sufficient blood/oxygen to the brain.

Testing for this will include an EKG and a treadmill stress test. Because many athletes already have some abnormal EKG findings while they are at rest, which could give us false findings in conjunction with a stress test, we recommend their stress test also includes some kind of imaging. This can be echocardiogram or nuclear imaging.

If the results are borderline and we are still not certain what is occurring, the next test should be a cardiac MRI to look at other causes of chest pain in these athletes.

Between all these tests, we should be able to determine the cause of the heart symptoms.

An Example

As the team cardiologist for the Sacramento Republic FC professional soccer team, I attended to one of the players who tried to do a bicycle kick in a game (where you kick a ball already in the air in a rearward direction) and fell hard on his back. He could not breathe at first, seemed to recover, and continued playing. He then had severe chest pains. Testing was done in the emergency room, and nothing of significance was found. Yet every time he exercised, he experienced chest pain.

They wanted me to clear his return to play. I waited a week and performed a stress test, which was normal. By this time, the symptoms had gone away. So most likely it was costochondritis (the inflammatory joint pain where cartilage attaches to ribs), or a rib trauma from falling so hard on his back and affecting his heart. You can sometimes have heart contusion from being hit in the chest.

Exertional Fatigue and Performance Decline

Two other categories of symptoms that can occur in athletes are worth mentioning.

One is *exertional fatigue*, in which an athlete complains of feeling more fatigued than normal while exercising. The other is *performance decline*, where they are unable to perform at the same intensity level as previously due to now more quickly becoming fatigued or experiencing shortness of breath.

For patients with either of these symptoms, an EKG should be performed. It is more likely to reveal these abnormalities in athletes under thirty-five. Because the underlying cause in athletes over thirty-five is more likely to be coronary disease, the baseline EKGs would not be helpful.

A treadmill test should be administered so the cardiologist can look further into the probable cause.

We should also check their oxygen saturation. If the saturation drops, they could have a congenital heart issue (such as a hole in the heart).

Shortness of Breath

If shortness of breath is one of a patient's symptoms (and they had not experienced this previously), we need to explore if it might be related to the heart or the lung. Or if something else entirely is occurring.

One way to assess this is by asking the patient, "When you experience shortness of breath, are you wheezing as well?" In that case, it could be due to exercise-induced asthma. If pulmonary function testing shows this to be the case, the patient can use an inhaler.

If the shortness of breath is *cardiac related*, the cause may depend on whether the patient is younger or older than thirty-five. If younger, the culprit may be inherited cardiovascular disorders (genetic), some of which we have described before. These can include hypertrophic cardiomyopathy (abnormal thickening of heart muscle in the left ventricle), or arrhythmogenic right ventricular dysplasia (where muscle tissue in the *right ventricle* is replaced by fat and/or scar tissue, causing arrhythmias, long QT syndrome / problems with the heart's electrical system).

If the patient is over thirty-five, the most common cause is blockages in their arteries.

Other Possible Causes

Shortness of breath can also be *unrelated* to the heart or lungs. Instead, it can be caused by the following:

- *Anemia*—the most common source, it is a condition that occurs when blood has insufficient amounts of hemoglobin (the portion of red blood cells that carries oxygen). I have treated very fit female athletes who have excessive bleeding during their periods, such that they are shorter of breath during that time and the following week. If you suspect you have anemia, have your doctor test your blood. If it confirms anemia, the doctor will likely advise iron supplementation along with blood testing to monitor your levels.
- *Autoimmune disease*—such as *scleroderma*, which affects the skin and/or other organs. Effects ultimately can range from very mild to life-threatening. Or *lupus*, which can affect numerous body systems, such as connective tissue, kidneys, joints, brain, lungs, or heart.
- *Infection*—the most common being mononucleosis (more frequent in younger people).
- *Hormonal problems*—especially thyroid issues.

Some of these conditions can be very serious, which is another reason to alert your doctor if you are experiencing shortness of breath as it may be a valuable clue to discovering an ailment that is best detected early.

Pay Attention

As you can see, even if you are an athlete in excellent physical shape, you are not exempt from ailments. If symptoms occur, do not pretend they are not happening or hide them. They serve an important purpose as they often are signs of an underlying condition that needs to be investigated and possibly treated.

No race or training routine is worth your life.

CHAPTER 11

HYPERTENSION IN ATHLETES

Despite a common belief that elevated blood pressure is usually associated with the middle-aged and older populations, hypertension is the most common cardiovascular condition in competitive athletes. In fact, high blood pressure issues are becoming increasingly prevalent overall. While I am not seeing an increase in the older population from what we have always had, I am finding more and more younger patients with hypertension.

In the United States, the prevalence in men ages twenty to twenty-nine overall (not just athletes) for hypertension is 14.4 percent. For females of this age range, the frequency is 6.2 percent. Numbers rise from there to 21 percent for men ages thirty to thirty-nine and to 10 percent in women.

Over the three decades I have been in the field (medical school 1989–1994, residency 1994–2000, private practice and academics 2000–2021), I have seen a significant surge in young people referred to my office with hypertension, particularly younger athletes. Whether they are taking performance-enhancing drugs or energy boosters or something else, these competitive athletes are in some way accelerating the rate of occurrence.

At the other end of the fitness scale, I am also seeing more younger hypertensive *nonathletes* who are overweight and taking weight-loss medications, such as the ephedrine type of stimulants or caffeine. Even though ephedrine is banned from over-the-counter sports and diet supplements, it is available by prescription (often as treatment for allergic disorders like bronchial asthma). People can also purchase certain combinations of over-the-counter drugs that, if taken jointly, would be comparable to ephedrine.

What Is Normal Blood Pressure?

One might ask, "What is the sweet spot for blood pressure in a well-oiled engine?"

Personally, I see the best as a systolic of 115 to 120 and diastolic of 75 to 80. In fact, studies have shown that with every twenty millimeters increase in systolic blood pressure (such as 115 to 135) or ten millimeters increase in diastolic pressure (such as 75 to 85), you double your risk of major cardiovascular event such as heart attack or stroke.

As a result, the American Heart Association and American College of Cardiology recently changed the criteria for hypertension so that people will be more alert to its seriousness and get treated sooner. Hypertension previously was said to be present when blood pressure was 140/90.

Now 130/80 is considered hypertensive.

Another change is that it had been thought that older individuals, such as those in their sixties and seventies, could have higher numbers without being considered hypertensive, but that has changed too.

Now above 130/80 is deemed hypertension for *everyone*.

(For those under the age of eighteen, we look at additional criteria of their age, height, and gender.)

Getting Accurate Readings

Unfortunately, offices of some general practitioner physicians may not know how to properly diagnose patients with hypertension, especially athletes. To get accurate BP readings, these protocols should be followed by the patient:

- Avoid caffeine, smoking, or exercise thirty minutes before checking the pressure as these can raise it.
- If you have a full bladder, empty it, as this can also raise blood pressure.
- When checking blood pressure, make sure your arm is at the same level as the heart. Not higher or lower.
- Rest (sit) for five minutes before checking.
- Test on both arms, as some people may have blockages in the arteries in one arm that can falsely show abnormal pressure. Take the measurement in each arm, with the higher number accepted as the correct blood pressure. Then wait two minutes and take the blood pressure again in the more accurate arm (that with the higher number) and average the two readings to determine your blood pressure.
- Two blood pressure checks are performed following these methods on two separate office visits.

White Coat Hypertension

While important for patients to know the numbers associated with high blood pressure, it is also valuable to realize that not *all* elevated measurements accurately point toward hypertension. At least not in the presence of a doctor, ironically.

White coat hypertension refers to patients having artificially elevated blood pressure when tested in the (white coated) doctor's office due to increased anxiety. This affects 15 percent of people.

On those occasions, when we get a high reading at our office, and the patient counterclaims the numbers are normal when measured on their own device at home, we typically have them wear an ambulatory blood pressure monitor to confirm it. The device automatically measures their BP every thirty to sixty minutes over a twenty-four-hour period. If we confirm their blood pressure is low outside of the office and high in the office, we conclude they have white coat hypertension and do not need to be treated.

Masked Hypertension

The flipside of this condition is something called *masked hypertension.* This describes a patient who has normal blood pressure when measured in the office but may have *nighttime hypertension.* We suspect this in patients when they present normal blood pressure in the office but have cardiovascular risk factors such as diabetes, obesity, a positive family history of heart disease, or high cholesterol. We also will consider this if they have symptoms of *end organ damage.*

End organ damage?

The threat from high blood pressure is not limited to the heart. Hypertension can also damage other end organs such as the kidneys, eyes, and brain, as the elevated pressure will eventually injure the small capillaries in these organs. Yet most patients do not notice any symptoms of their high blood pressure. That is why hypertension is called the silent killer.

So even if we measure normal blood pressure in the office, if the patient shows these other risk factors, we have them wear an ambulatory blood pressure monitor. Another indicator for conducting this further study is protein in the urine, since once hypertension has damaged the capillaries in kidneys, they start spilling protein. Or if an eye exam shows changes in the little capillaries in the eye. Or if a carotenoid ultrasound shows plaque formation in the arteries.

Using the Ambulatory Blood Pressure Monitor

An ambulatory blood pressure monitor automatically takes a patient's blood pressure measurement every thirty to sixty minutes for twenty-four hours, resulting in a graph for the physician to read when the patient returns the monitor the next day.

Regrettably, most doctors, including most cardiologists, do not use an ambulatory monitor. This is not due to its lack of effectiveness; rather, it comes down to economy. It is very difficult to be reimbursed for this by insurance. Yet it can yield important information, and insurance companies would be wise to consider better coverage of its use.

For instance, when we sleep at night, our blood pressure normally drops by 10 percent. This is called *dipping*. But if someone has *nocturnal hypertension*, their blood pressure does not drop at night. This has been shown to result in higher cardiovascular mortality.

When we see patients with nocturnal hypertension, and their pressure is *higher than normal* at night, we consider other disease states that could cause this elevated pressure. One possibility is obstructive sleep apnea. Or untreated hyperthyroid disease. Or kidney disease. Or a tumor that can raise aldosterone hormone, which regulates sodium balance, blood volume, and blood pressure. All issues that should be addressed.

Clearly, an ambulatory monitor can be a very valuable diagnostic tool!

It should be noted that the criteria for diagnosing hypertension with an ambulatory monitor is somewhat different than in the office setting. For nonathletes, the average for all the blood pressure measurements by an ambulatory monitor (which includes the patient standing, moving, eating, etc.) is considered normal when the normal average daytime blood pressure would need be 135/85 or less and nighttime blood pressure of 120/70 or smaller. Anything above these amounts would be indicative of hypertension.

For athletes, we want to do additional testing.

Since athletes participate in strenuous physical activities, we do a treadmill stress test to see if they have exaggerated (during exercise) response in blood pressure. As we conduct this exercise test, systolic blood pressure should not go above 200 to 210 in males and not over 190 in females. If it exceeds those numbers (even in patients whose blood pressure is normal or borderline at rest), we conclude there is *exaggerated hypertension* that needs to be treated.

Furthermore, even if blood pressure does not exceed those numbers during the exercise portion of the test, once the exertion ends and they enter a period of recovery, their BP should move lower than 140/90 within five minutes. If it does not, we again conclude there is a hypertension issue.

Hypertension Diagnosis Triggers Need for Other Tests

If the patient is believed to have hypertension, an EKG should be administered. This is done to look for any end organ changes in the heart, since with hypertension, the heart has to squeeze against the elevated pressure and can become thickened (hypertrophic). It is also important the patient have a full blood panel that includes a cholesterol check.

If your doctor (general practitioner or cardiologist) does not suggest both of these, *it is up to the patient to insist.*

The truth is, I perform an EKG on any patient that is referred to my office.

Populations More Prone to Hypertension

While everyone is susceptible to hypertension, some groups of people are especially disposed to the disease.

Generally, more males suffer from high blood pressure than females, though both sexes have a greater likelihood to develop hypertension as they age, as do individuals who are overweight.

African Americans have a higher prevalence of hypertension because of their genetics. They also tend to have more severe hypertension and exhibit it at an earlier age. Furthermore, African Americans are more prone to strokes and kidney disease as a result of high blood pressure.

Thus, people in susceptible groups are especially encouraged to establish health habits that diminish their chances of developing hypertension.

Why Hypertension in Athletes?

To answer the question of why an increasing prevalence of high blood pressure is occurring in the very group that is expected to be healthiest (athletes), we must address the unique situation that can apply to those who are very physically active.

I often repeat the fact that knowing the family's medical history is extremely important in treating a patient. This is certainly true when it comes to hypertension and particularly for the athlete patient.

If you have a negative family history of hypertension, and you have normal blood pressure, athletic exercise will remodel the heart *eccentrically*. That means the heart muscle can thicken over time but only in certain areas. This is actually beneficial as the heart becomes more efficient when it squeezes and relaxes. It now can pump the same amount of blood to the rest of the body in one heartbeat that otherwise might have required four beats. This is why the heart rates of athletes tend to be lower, especially at rest, since their heart function becomes more effective.

However, it was recently discovered that if you have a *positive family history of hypertension*, when your heart remodels from athletic exercise, it does so *concentrically*. That means the muscle *all around the heart* thickens. This makes the heart very stiff, such that it does not adequately relax to fill up with sufficient blood during the beating process.

So if an athlete does have a family history of hypertension, chances are that exercise will cause the heart to remodel in a negative fashion. Fortunately, all the benefits of exercise will still outweigh this issue.

But that counterbalance is lost if the athlete has high blood pressure.

Since hypertension *itself* can make a heart thicken over time, those athletes *also* having a family history of hypertension (which tends to cause hearts to thicken overall from exercise) have to be even more careful. They need to be all the more aggressive in lowering their blood pressure.

Gaining Competitive Advantage = Blood Pressure Problems

But there is another reason that athletes in particular may experience hypertension. To understand this, we first must point out that there are two types of high blood pressure: *primary hypertension* and *secondary hypertension*.

Primary hypertension is the result of how a person's intrinsic biology and anatomy functions. This accounts for 90 percent of cases of high blood pressure.

But 10 percent of hypertensive patients have what we call *secondary hypertension*. Secondary hypertension has outside contributing factors, including some that athletes may engage in to become more competitive. Likely outside influences could be the following:

- PEDs (performance-enhancing drugs) or PES (performance-enhancing substances). These can include growth hormones or erythropoietin (to stimulate production of more red blood cells that increases the blood's oxygen-carrying capacity).
- Some athletes, like linebackers in football, increase their eating to gain weight and become bigger to better block running backs, etc.
- Nonsteroidal anti-inflammatory drugs like Motrin and Naprosyn, often used by athletes to cope with injuries and strains, can affect kidneys and raise blood pressure.
- Anergic hormones, such as catecholamines (stress hormones).
- Additionally, athletes may incur injuries causing pain, and pain can raise blood pressure.

Our bodies are finely tuned machines. That is why when we add substances to it, there are usually side effects.

Any of these above actions can contribute to a rise in blood pressure. In other words, if we were to simply withdraw these outside inducements, the affected athlete's blood pressure could be normal.

Looking Beyond the Obvious

Typically, young people should not have hypertension. Anytime a patient under thirty years old comes in with that diagnosis, and no family history of high blood pressure or other obvious causes (such as obesity), I look for nontypical causes of hypertension.

If a patient (any age) has *very* high blood pressure, above 180/100, I particularly want to check if they have *secondary* hypertension. The same is true if they are already on three different blood pressure medications and still have high blood pressure, as something else may be occurring beyond the blood pressure issue.

Additional scrutiny is also necessary if I have someone wear an ambulatory blood pressure monitor and their BP does not dip at night as it should. Or if a patient I have been treating who has been exhibiting normal blood pressure because of treatment suddenly has their pressure shoot up.

These red flags should tip off doctors catering to both the general populace and athletes that something is wrong, and other causes need to be ruled out. Further examination can include a urine test, comprehensive blood test that includes a metanephrines test, and cortisol (stress hormone) level test. We are looking for indications of some other disease issue elevating the blood pressure.

Kidneys Raising Blood Pressure

An example of BP rising due to an issue in another organ is when there is a narrowing (stenosis) in the renal arteries that carry blood to the kidneys.

In young people, this narrowing is due to fibromuscular dysplasia, a genetic condition/predisposition that causes muscles around the arteries to thicken, which in turn narrows the renal arteries. This results in less blood flow to the kidneys. When this decrease in blood flow occurs, the kidneys respond as if there must be bleeding somewhere in the body causing this reduction in the blood traveling to the kidneys. The kidneys turn on the RAAS system (renin-angiotensin-aldosterone system). This is a critical regulator of blood volume and systemic vascular resistance, which together affect cardiac output and arterial pressure (blood pressure). Through these mechanisms, the body can elevate the blood pressure in a prolonged manner.

In this case, hypertension is due to a problem in the arteries to the kidneys. If diagnosed and treated with the insertion of a stent to keep the renal arteries open, the patient's hypertension is eliminated.

Now, if an ultrasound in an older person shows narrowing of these renal arteries, the cause is usually fat buildup. It still leads to the same problem (activated RAAS system) and elevated blood pressure. Insertion of a stent again opens up the artery, deactivates the RAAS system, and returns the blood pressure to normal. So even with a fat deposit, a stent is the solution.

Stimulants to Avoid for Patients Diagnosed with Hypertension

All patients, athletes and nonathletes, who have been diagnosed with hypertension, should avoid stimulants that can elevate blood pressure. These include the following:

- Coffee
- Energy drinks
- Amphetamines
- Ephedrine
- Smoking
- Alcohol
- Herbs that may aggravate high blood pressure such as guarana and licorice (includes licorice as both candy and supplement)
- Blood pressure can also rise from ingestion of:
- Anabolic steroids (taken to build up muscles)
- Some antidepressants
- Diet pills

Additionally, all people with high blood pressure should avoid nonsteroidal anti-inflammatory NSAIDs such as Advil and Motrin. If there is pain, patients are better served using Tylenol.

Women should also be aware that if they begin taking oral contraceptives, they have a 5 percent higher chance of developing hypertension within five years.

Treating Hypertension without Medication

The treatment of hypertension offers two primary approaches: non-pharmacological and pharmacological (drugs).

Nonpharmacological treatment is best reserved for those people who have only borderline hypertension (systolic hovering near 130) and there are no signs of target organ damage (an EKG indicates normal heart muscle, an eye exam shows no abnormality, and kidney function is good).

Nonpharmacological steps include:

- Reducing weight
- Reducing intake of salt/sodium significantly
- Ceasing smoking
- Ceasing intake of alcohol
- Ceasing intake of coffee
- Ceasing intake of energy stimulants
- Ceasing use of performance-enhancing substances

As you can see, all the above examples relate to what *we put in* our bodies, as this always has an immense influence on our health. This brings us to one of the most significant arenas in managing hypertension: choosing the foods we eat.

Healthy Diet

In addition to the above behavioral changes, there are two diets that are very helpful: the Mediterranean diet and the Dietary Approaches to Stop Hypertension (DASH) diet.

No matter how much you exercise, you cannot assume your level of activity compensates for eating fatty high-cholesterol salty foods or having a family history for heart attacks.

A friend of mine on the management side of professional sports exercised regularly. Yet he once was jogging in Seattle and developed chest pains. He wisely stopped and had himself checked. Turned out he had a critical blockage. A stent was put in, and he has been exercising without issue ever since.

Exercise certainly reduces chances for a cardiac event (and may have helped prevent my friend from having a heart attack). But even marathon runners and others who exercise intensely can end up dying because they are not eating well, thinking they are immune to the effects of poor dietary habits. They are not.

The Mediterranean diet is a healthy approach to eating and has been shown to reduce cardiovascular mortality and morbidity, lower breast cancer in women, as well as lessen risk of Alzheimer's and Parkinson's.

The essentials of this diet are as follows:

- Increased intake of plant-based foods
- Fish or chicken for protein
- Olive oil as substitute for butter
- Herbs instead of salt
- Nuts (a good source of linoleic acid, a type of the omega-3 fatty acids also found in fish that lowers triglycerides and blood pressure, improves health of the vessels, and reduces chances of blood clots and sudden cardiac death)

When I was younger, a couple of colleagues and I visited Spain. In addition to enjoying meals that reflected this Mediterranean diet, our visit was enlightening as we discovered aspects of their lifestyle much different from ours in the United States. Including some that might offer added health benefits.

After arriving, we began our stay there in vacation mode, sleeping in during the morning and then going out for a late breakfast, only to discover all the restaurants and stores were closed! We wondered where everyone was. Was it a holiday?

No, it was siesta.

Siestas are a long-established tradition where people go home to have a big lunch in the afternoon and sleep. Interestingly, recent research has shown that if you get twenty minutes of a power nap (and not more than twenty minutes) in the afternoon, it can lower your chances for cardiovascular disease as the stress hormone cortisol is reduced during an afternoon nap.

At 5:00 p.m., everyone returns to work until nine. Then a light dinner, after which people go out for a walk that burns off calories, which in addition to their Mediterranean diet, helps them have less cardiovascular complications than in the United States.

DASH

The DASH diet is the Americanized version of the Mediterranean diet. NIH (National Institutes of Health) research has shown that the DASH diet not only lowers blood pressure but also lessens incidences of cancer, stroke, heart failure, diabetes, as well as reduces cholesterol.

Similar to the Mediterranean diet, the DASH diet includes daily:

- At least four servings of fruit and vegetables
- Two to four servings of low-fat and non-fat dairy products
- At least one serving of nuts, beans, or seeds
- One and a half to two servings of lean meats, fish, or poultry
- Limits on fats and sweets as much as possible

Note: There are two other variations of the DASH diet, which include a weight-loss plan as well as a vegetarian plan.

Exercise

Exercise is the other nonpharmacological treatment for hypertension.

If patients are prehypertensive (systolic blood pressure between 115 and 130), dynamic resistance exercise may be slightly the better choice for exercise. These would include pushups, sit-ups, squat thrusts, step-ups, and weightlifting.

Isometric exercise is helpful for *all* patients, regardless of whether they have prehypertension or hypertension. This is strength training in static postures where you do not lengthen the muscle. An example is the plank, in which the body is held in a position similar to a pushup, but supported on the forearms rather than hands.

If a patient has already been diagnosed with hypertension, moderate endurance exercise such as jogging for extended periods is the best type of activity.

Even regular brisk walking is helpful and recommended for those unable to participate in more active pursuits.

Interestingly, increasing from moderate to *vigorous* physical activity does *not* reduce blood pressure any further. So patients do not need to feel compelled to overdo workouts to lower blood pressure. Routine moderate exercise, five days a week, will give all the benefits that exercise can offer.

This is also why competitive athletes do not have an advantage over others to lower their blood pressure. While we might presume their heightened levels of physical activity would further decrease blood pressure, we find it has no added benefits over the moderate exercise available to most noncompetitors.

Also, please note that more vigorous aerobic cardiovascular exercise, such as running and swimming, only reduces daytime blood pressure, not nighttime blood pressure (as during sleep).

Pharmacological Treatment

As said, nonpharmacological treatment is best for people with only borderline hypertension (systolic hovering near 130) and no signs of target organ damage. But if you have hypertension, or even if you have borderline hypertension and there are any signs of target organ damage or there is a high cardiovascular risk score, you want to treat pharmacologically.

My website's Resources page has the Framingham Heart Risk score calculator, where you can input your age, cholesterol level, gender, weight, and other factors, and it tells what your risk of heart attack or stroke would be during the next ten years. Less than 5 percent is considered low risk, above 7.5 is intermediate risk, while over 20 percent is high risk. If you have a high-risk cardiovascular score, you should take medication even if your blood pressure is borderline hypertensive.

Calculated 10-Year Risk	Risk Category
Less than 5%	Low
5% to 7.4%	Borderline
7.5% to 19.9%	Intermediate
Greater than 20%	High

Cardiac Risk Assessment

Many people, especially those without extreme hypertension or obvious heart risk factors, may be getting treated by their primary care doctors. It is especially important for these patients to know how to be proactive in their care since many general practitioner doctors unfortunately do not know how to properly treat hypertension, including those borderline cases, with regard to when to focus on diet or when to start medication or which medication.

Other Considerations: Gender, Age, and Ethnicity

Further factors in the proper selection of heart medications include the patient's gender and age and possibly ethnicity.

There are commonly prescribed classes of drugs called ACE inhibitors (angiotensin converting enzyme inhibitors) or ARB (angiotensin II receptor blockers). But we do not want to use either of these in young females because if they get pregnant, these drugs can negatively affect kidney development in the embryo. Fortunately, other types of drugs are safe during pregnancy, specifically beta-blockers (beta-adrenergic blocking agents) like labetalol or non-beta-blockers like methyldopa.

Different drugs are prescribed for African Americans and non-African Americans because of differing genetic makeups. African Americans do not respond well to ACE inhibitors (which tend to cause allergic reactions called angioedema that make the mouth and throat swell up) or to beta-blockers. I recently treated a hypertensive African American running back on a local high school's football team. An elite athlete, he was to attend one of the country's premier universities to play on their team. We started him on a calcium channel blocker (such as Amlodipine), as this safely dilates (opens up) vessels without affecting the kidneys and is effective in African Americans (who tend to have salt-sensitive hypertension). If a patient's blood pressure does not lower to the target numbers with this, we can then add a diuretic class drug for African Americans.

Note that I am only giving general guidelines here, as we aspire to fine-tune the drug selection for each patient, as every individual responds to treatment differently.

Hypertensive Athlete Resuming Activity

Once a patient is receiving treatment (diagnosis is determined, the patient is improving their diet and committed to moderate exercise, along with medications taken if appropriate), they will ask the physician, "Doc, when can I jump back in and continue my sport?"

The answer would be "If you only have prehypertension or borderline high blood pressure, then you do not have any restriction. But if you have hypertension and an echocardiogram shows thickening of the heart muscle [hypertrophic cardiomyopathy], even if you have begun medication, you must immediately stop any *rigorous exercise*. That is categorized in sports medicine as very active category 3 and 3c sports, such as basketball, competitive swimming, soccer, football, racquetball [see chart below]. However, as soon as we measure, in the office, that blood pressure has been normal on two separate occasions, then we can clear you to return to your vigorous activity."

Positive Forecast!

While a diagnosis of high blood pressure is never welcome, patients can be comforted that the medical field today, in conjunction with the individual adjusting their habits, has numerous ways to successfully treat this condition and keep it under control in both athletes and nonathletes.

CHAPTER 12

ATRIAL FIBRILLATION IN ATHLETES

Arrhythmias are irregular heartbeats. This can be a heart that beats too fast or too slow or beats in an abnormal pattern.

As the most common form of arrhythmia, atrial fibrillation is estimated to affect thirty-three million people worldwide. Hypertension and age increase the risk for having this condition. While there is a 1.5 percent prevalence for someone in their fifties to experience it, that increases to 20 percent for those over the age of eighty-five.

As we will see, *a particular extreme athletic activity can also cause it.* So how serious is it?

Arrhythmias are divided into supraventricular (meaning *above the ventricle,* in the left or right atrium) or ventricular (in left or right ventricle). Supraventricular (in an atrium) are usually not fatal. But *ventricular arrhythmias* can cause death—most commonly when in the left ventricle—as that pumps blood to the brain and the rest of the body. (The right ventricle pumps blood to the lungs.)

Some atrial fibrillations can occur and then spontaneously go back to a normal heart rhythm (called *paroxysmal,* meaning starts and stops). But AFib can also continue without returning to normal (*persistent* atrial fibrillation). If physicians are unable to return AFib to normal, and this condition continues over a year, it is termed *chronic.*

What Is Atrial Fibrillation?

Let us start with this important question: How does a heart beat?

An electrical impulse is generated from the sinus node (also known as the SA node) in the wall of the right atrium, near the top of the heart.

This impulse first causes the atrium to beat.

The impulse then continues to travel down electrical pathways in the heart to the atrioventricular node (AV node). The AV node is a circular structure of fibers *between* the atrium and the ventricle. It regulates the flow of electricity from the top of the heart to the bottom (from atrium to ventricle).

The AV node then distributes electrical impulses to the left and right ventricles. It does this through two bundles of nerves (conveniently called the left bundle and right bundle). The two ventricles squeeze simultaneously.

So now the heart has beat properly from top to bottom, maintaining the natural pumping action to effectively oxygenate the whole body.

But with atrial fibrillation, the atrium begins *fibrillating* (a quivering movement due to uncoordinated contractions). The heart no longer squeezes. Instead, it sort of shivers.

Why does this happen?

Instead of responding to the electrical impulses that are naturally generated in the heart, some muscle cells start firing on their own. In fact, so many cells can be firing simultaneously that the heart rate can be between 400 to 500 beats per minute.

When these rapid impulses travel down to the AV node, they get slowed somewhat, so that by the time they reach the ventricles, the heart rate can be between 80 to 200 *and* very irregular. Normally, there is only one impulse at a time traveling from the atrium to the ventricle. But if so many cells are firing, sending impulses down toward the ventricle, the AV node gets overworked. It cannot filter out most of these extra impulses. So many of these electrical signals get through, causing the ventricle to pump rapidly, most commonly around 150 beats per minute (for people with healthy AV nodes).

This is when patients experience symptoms, because the heartbeat is fast and irregular. The ventricle does not have enough time to fill with blood from the atrium, so the ventricle does not pump out sufficient blood. This can also cause pressure in the left atrium to increase, such that fluid gets pushed into the alveoli in the lungs and can lead to significant shortness of breath.

Atrial Fibrillation Symptoms

How can you know if you have atrial fibrillation?

The symptoms may vary greatly from person to person. Some people will not feel much, while others experience extreme tiredness. Some feel light-headed (too little blood going to the brain) to the point that they may pass out. But the most common symptoms are palpitations (feeling your heart is beating too fast, skipping beats, or fluttering) and fatigue.

Yet there can be more serious symptoms as well.

When someone is diagnosed with atrial fibrillation, doctors are concerned with two things. The first goal is to slow down the heart rate. The second concern is clotting. Since an atrium experiencing atrial fibrillation is shivering rather than squeezing, blood inside the atrium is not leaving as it normally would. It is instead being shaken, and that blood can clot together. Unfortunately, that clotted blood can then travel into the ventricle and be pumped out into the body, causing serious problems, including a major stroke if it settles in the brain.

Causes of Atrial Fibrillation

The most common cause of atrial fibrillation is hypertension. Other causes can include obesity and obstructive sleep apnea. Interestingly, very tall people are more prone to this condition than shorter people.

Yet there is an additional cause that most people are not aware of: exercise.

Specifically, one type of exercise.

Marathons

Until now, we have focused on the many ways that exercise is good for you. However, extreme endurance exercise such as marathons, be they running, swimming, and/or biking, can increase the chances of developing atrial fibrillation *years later*.

This came to light from a study of those who ran in the 1992 Barcelona marathon. Tracking these people eleven years later, the study found that participants had an 8.8 times increased risk of developing atrial fibrillation compared to people who do not run marathons.

While they are not entirely sure why atrial fibrillation occurs, there are hypotheses. It is known that people who train for and run marathons come down with the flu more often, since the sustained physical exertion is such a strain on the body that it suppresses the immune system. Some researchers believe this suppression of the immune system also leads to chronic inflammation around the atrium. This can result in fibrosis or scarring in the heart, which can later trigger atrial fibrillation.

In fact, when EKGs are done on atrial fibrillation patients, the P-wave is prolonged, which correlates with irregular contraction of the atrium and usually means fibrosis, something that is seen in endurance athletes.

The other hypothesis is when people exercise, there is a transient (temporary) enlargement in the left atrium, and that stretches the atrium. This increases the mass of the atrium, which can lead to atrial fibrillation in the future.

Delayed Occurrence

In endurance athletes, atrial fibrillation most commonly happens between ages forty to sixty, even after many of these people are no longer running marathons. It does not occur while they are younger because the condition takes time to emerge (it usually takes a minimum of ten years to develop the scarring and fibrosis).

While I do not wish to deter those who want to run a marathon, I feel it necessary to point out these documented links between the extreme exercise and atrial fibrillation. This cause and effect has been documented in animal studies but not yet in humans. But we do see evidence of this condition occurring, as in the study showing that Barcelona marathoners had an almost ninefold greater chance of developing AFib later.

This awareness is critically important for those who undertake such exercise. As more and more people are running marathons around the world, the expectation is the incidence of AFib is likewise going to increase. However, since athletes are normally in very good health overall, they may not *notice* the typical effects of atrial fibrillation as quickly as the average person.

However, there is one negative effect that will be highly perceptible to the athlete.

When an atrium is functioning well, there is an atrial kick that moves more blood into the ventricle during the last portion of the ventricle's filling cycle. The ventricle then sends more blood into the body. But that atrial kick is gone with atrial fibrillation, as athletes lose about 40 percent of their left ventricle filling ability. The obvious result is the athlete cannot perform as well as they normally would.

Can Happen at Unexpected Times

Atrial fibrillation may also occur during a time when you think it would be most unlikely. At least in athletes.

Our bodies have an autonomic nervous system that controls the body's involuntary functions. It is composed of two divisions. One is the sympathetic nervous system that *speeds up our responses*, as if to a perceived threat (triggering our fight-or-flight reaction) or when we simply *are physically active*. There is also the parasympathetic system, which controls the body *while at rest*.

The sympathetic nervous system's release of stress hormones to speed up body responses, such as when we are fearful, angry, or exercising, can cause arrhythmias, since atrial fibrillation is a fast rhythm.

Yet in athletes, atrial fibrillation *can also occur* when the parasympathetic nervous system engages to slow things down.

Why? The heart rate in athletes is often already slow, but when they are sleeping or after big meals, the parasympathetic system still kicks in to slow things down further. *That* can trigger AFib in athletes. Again, this is less likely to occur in young athletes but can unexpectedly surface years later. Athletes (or ex-athletes) should be alert to this, so if they feel palpitations during or after sleep or after a big meal, they need to realize it could be atrial fibrillation and should get their heart checked.

Moderate Exercise = Decreased Risk

A useful way to look at maintaining health is that our body functions best in moderation. A balance. If there is too much of one thing, there will be an imbalance in other areas.

Moderation is how we should also live our lives. If we are too extreme in any area, it can throw us off in other arenas. For example, if your lifestyle is causing you to be in a fight-or-flight state too often, you can develop chronic stress or anxiety, which can harm your health. At the same time, if we are too relaxed, living a life with little activity (too sedentary), that imbalances our natural system as well.

Unlike the increased risk associated with extreme exercise, research has found decreased risk for atrial fibrillation for those who do moderate exercise. This decrease also applies to older adults that exercise moderately.

The reason? Regular moderate exercise reduces chances of developing high blood pressure or coronary artery disease that contribute to the likelihood of atrial fibrillation.

Ruling Out Secondary Causes

With any atrial fibrillation, we first want to rule out secondary causes, such as thyroid disease, which is tested for through blood work. We also want to rule out that the patient is taking performance-enhancing drugs that might cause AFib. Or that there may be some types of tumors releasing stress hormones.

Treatments

There are two approaches to treating AFib.

Interventional cardiologists like myself may shock the heart using a defibrillator to reset the rhythm, a process then followed by medication. This is the most common way to restore a proper heartbeat. I have done thousands of these on patients.

There are also electrical specialists called EP doctors (electrophysiologists), who can direct a catheter up through the groin artery to locate the cause in the atrium. It is almost always near where the four pulmonary veins deliver blood into the atrium. Once they find the area of bad cells most responsible for triggering the other cells and causing AFib, these doctors perform *ablation*, that is, they burn this area.

The cure rate is low for this approach, about 40 percent. But when ablations work, patients are cured in that they will most likely not develop atrial fibrillation again. Plus, in general, ablations may be desirable as the procedure does not have side effects, nor most of the time require follow-up medication. But it does involve more risk. Anytime you enter the heart to burn muscle cells, there is a chance you may puncture the heart.

Choosing the Right Treatment

If the athlete says they will no longer perform competitive sports and instead continue with moderate exercise, we may let them stay in AFib and simply take medications to control their heart rate so it does not go above 100 (such as when exercising or stressing). Or we can more aggressively work on returning the heart rhythm back to normal with shocking and medication.

Older studies had indicated these two were equal choices for patients: Using only medication to control the heart rate yielded the same benefits as shocking the patient to return their normal rhythm. But more recent studies now indicate that restoring a normal sinus rhythm in patients by shocking is better.

However, one should not wait too long to correct this issue. Numerous times, patients have come to me that were treated by others and have had AFib for over a year. But if patients have been in AFib for over one year, it becomes difficult to correct. By that point, the problematic cells alter form. There is more scarring, and the atrium enlarges. The success rate of ablation on them becomes extremely low as well.

If a patient's atrium has enlarged to over 50 mm, or they have been in AFib for over a year, then their only realistic choice is to go on heart rate-controlling medications.

So the guidance here is like with nearly every medical condition: the earlier that AFib is treated, the better.

Alternatively, if the patient wants to continue participating in competitive sports, neither of these last two options is the right one. On the other hand, if the AFib in an athlete is well tolerated and not that frequent, then the athlete can fully participate in competition and exercise. This also means we cannot shock them, as that always requires follow-up medication to continue as well.

In such cases, we would send the patient to an EP specialist for ablations.

Medications

There are different anti-arrhythmic drugs available, classified based on their mechanism of action. They are designated as class 1, class 2, or class 3.

A class 1 drug would be used if someone has infrequent symptoms, such as atrial fibrillation only once every month or two when exercising. The patient carries the medication with them and takes it whenever they get symptoms in order to settle it down. Literally called the pill-in-the-pocket approach, this is often used in sports cardiology. The two drugs recommended for this would be Propafenone and Flecainide.

Class 2 drugs are not given for atrial fibrillation as those are used for ventricular tachycardia (having to do with the ventricle), not with atrium issues.

Class 3 drugs can be used for athletes having frequent symptoms, and while the medications do not have immediately noticeable acute side effects, they do have side effects if used for a long time. Such drugs are Amiodarone or Sotalol.

Years ago, there was a commonly prescribed drug called Digoxin. When I first began practicing, I was using it for people with atrial fibrillation or those with heart failure. But over the years, both my experience and scientific studies have shown this drug to have some toxicity and to cause increased mortality. As a result, Digoxin has fallen out of use. Athletes especially should avoid it as it is not effective when a person is exercising.

Separate from anti-arrhythmic-type drugs, we have medications that simply slow down the heart rate. Those are called calcium channel blockers, such as Cardizem or Deratamil, or beta-blockers, such as Lopressor or Inderal.

Anticoagulation Medication (Blood Thinners)

As noted earlier in this chapter, one of the risks with atrial fibrillation is blood clotting that can lead to a stroke. Cardiologists employ a specific method to determine which atrial fibrillation patients should be taking anticoagulation medication (blood thinners) to prevent clotting.

Called CHADS-VASc, this acronym's letters stand for the following risk factors:

> *C* for congestive heart failure
> *H* for hypertension
> *A* for age over seventy-five
> *D* for diabetes
> *S* for (prior) stroke
> *V* for vascular disease
> *A* for ages sixty-five to seventy-five
> *Sc* for the sex of the patient (females have a higher risk for strokes than males)

CHADS-VASc determines who we should anticoagulate based on a point system. If a patient has a condition described in any of these different categories, they get one point. The only exceptions to this are categories age over seventy-five or a prior stroke, which are each worth two points.

If someone's score is two or more, they should be anticoagulated. But if, for example, someone is simply over forty years old and has only hypertension, they only get one point, as their risk of developing blood clots is extremely low. Thus, they do not need to be on blood thinners.

Athletes are scored in the same way as nonathletes.

While a person can continue their physical activities while on blood thinners, we recommend they not continue any contact sports as that can cause bruising or bleeding, which can be serious for someone whose blood is not coagulating normally due to medication.

The bottom line for athletes (and nonathletes) is that while there is nothing they can do to prevent atrial fibrillation (beyond the avoidance of marathons or other extreme endurance sports or drinking alcohol or taking performance-enhancing drugs), they should pay particular attention to symptoms that may point to atrial fibrillation and report those to a physician. I will note studies have shown that long-distance competitive skiing is the sport associated with the highest risk of developing AFib. It also correlated to the number of events participated in a year and the duration of those events. The more events and the longer they last, the higher chance of developing AFib.

Better to Know Than Not, Reporting If You May Have AFib

I am sure there are people out there, perhaps some even reading this book, who may have at times suspected they have AFib, but since it is not interfering in their physical activity or daily life, have not reported it to their physician. That is not wise. In fact, in addition to being a possible risk to health, AFib can also inhibit the quality of one's life.

A patient in his sixties was sent to me by his primary doctor after it was determined he was in atrial fibrillation. The patient did not know it and would exercise all the time without any issues. In fact, he had been the athletic director for Stanford md and is the one who hired Bill Walsh as coach for Stanford, before Walsh was later hired by the San Francisco 49ers. After retiring from Stanford, he moved to my area and became athletic director at University of the Pacific.

Because he would exercise every day without symptoms, we had no idea how long he had been in AFib. Yet I shocked him, and he returned to a normal heart rhythm. He soon reported to me, "You know, even though I had atrial fibrillation, I never had symptoms and always felt great. But I have to tell you, ever since my normal rhythm returned, I have much more energy! I think much more clearly and do things more easily."

Unfortunately, after a week, his AFib returned. He even went to Stanford to get ablation, but it did not work. So he is now in AFib and taking blood thinners on a long-term basis. He is still exercising and feeling fine, but for that one week with normal sinus rhythm, he felt much better.

I mention this story because even if one is not experiencing dramatic symptoms from atrial fibrillation, it is possible that the quality of your life may improve if your heart can be returned to normal rhythm. Five percent of people in AFib do not even know it. But if you ever have symptoms that make you suspect you *might* have it, report that to your physician.

You may save, or even just improve, someone's life. Yours.

CHAPTER 13

ENDURANCE SPORTS

Extreme Sports, Beneficial or Harmful?

As you have read, exercise is fantastically beneficial for your body.

Until it's not.

There are certain levels of physical activity that, while demonstrating admirable personal commitment and achievement, may cause unanticipated harm.

Based on vast collected research, we know the *minimum* exercise needed to attain a wide range of benefits, from vascular health, to increased levels of concentration, to reducing specific cancer risks, Parkinson's, Alzheimer's, overall mortality, and more.

Less clear are the benefits and concerns about the other end of this spectrum: ultra-extreme sports.

Those activities that truly test the endurance, strength, and abilities of the participants. These include marathons (26-mile runs) and ultra-marathons (30- to 100-mile runs), cycling (over 75 miles), triathlons (commonly a 0.9-mile swim, 24.8-mile bicycle ride, and 26-mile run), and the Ironman Triathlon (2.4-mile swim, 112-mile bicycle ride, and 26-mile run).

The questions that come up are these: Is participating in such extreme sports more beneficial? Not beneficial? Or detrimental?

We certainly know that the hearts of endurance athletes can become very efficient. A normal person's heart rate is anywhere between fifty and one hundred beats per minute. Yet an endurance athlete can have a resting heart rate as low as thirty. That is because one pump of their heart can circulate more blood than what would be typical for someone who is not that caliber of an athlete. The endurance athlete has a higher stroke volume, an increase in the amount of blood pumped out for every heartbeat. A nonathlete may have a stroke volume of fifty to sixty milliliters per beat at rest. But an endurance athlete can have a stroke volume of ninety milliliter per beat at rest. That is why their heart can beat at only thirty beats per minute. They are pushing out so much more blood per beat. That also means their heart rate will not need to rise as high during exercise as would a nonathlete's for the same activity.

Considering all this, and what we already learned about the numerous exercise benefits, one might expect more intense exercise, requiring participants to be in even better physical condition would be more advantageous.

Many believe that to be the case.

But is it?

The Nature of Extreme Exercise

As addressed numerous times in this book, exercise is normally highly beneficial. The World Health Organization recommends 150 minutes per week of moderate exercise (walking or jogging between three to six miles per hour) or 75 minutes per week of vigorous exercise (over six miles per hour). This has been shown to reduce bad cholesterol (LDL) and raise good cholesterol (HDL) within three months. It also lowers blood pressure, incidence of obesity, the chance of metabolic syndrome (that leads to obesity), as well as stress.

While it should be emphasized again that people who have long been sedentary can be at a great health risk if they suddenly begin vigorous exercise, starting a properly paced exercise program based on your current condition has repeatedly been proven to produce positive results.

Unexpected Truth: the U-Shape

Yet surprisingly, research reveals something one might not anticipate. Even when someone undertakes an exercise regimen initially appropriate to their fitness level, as the duration and intensity of exercise grows greater, we encounter the U-shaped response.

Certainly as you exercise and reduce risks of heart attacks, strokes, etc., the rate of those risks follows the downward trend represented in the first descending leg of a U-shape.

But as exercise increases, it progresses to a point where the risks *start going back up,* shown in the upward direction of the second leg of the U. At that point, you are actually causing harm.

So the question becomes, What level of exercise is all you need to get all the benefits? When do you no longer need to do more?

How Much Is Enough?

A question I often hear from my patients: "What is the maximum amount of exercise I should do to get the most value?"

Fortunately, we have reports on studies that collectively looked at 416,175 healthy people over the age of twenty and tracked their exercise habits and health for eight years. The finding was that fifteen minutes per day of moderate exercise decreases all causes of mortality (not only cardiovascular) by 14 percent and increases life expectancy by three years. Then every added fifteen minutes of moderate exercise lowers all causes of mortality by an additional 4 percent.

Final Figures

Ultimately, they found people gained the most benefit toward decreasing all causes of mortality by doing one hundred minutes of moderate exercise, or fifty to sixty minutes of vigorous exercise, daily. There are no additional benefits to performing further exercise.

Yet these daily one hundred minutes moderate exercise or fifty to sixty minutes of vigorous exercise can reduce mortality by nearly 35 percent!

That, my friends, is huge.

While I am not yet aware of any definitive studies, I believe this desired level of exercise could extend one's lifespan by ten years.

Supportive Facts

Other studies also report highly positive conclusions, even when the study parameters and specific results vary from those mentioned above.

The Copenhagen City Heart Study (2015) looked at 1,878 runners/joggers versus 10,158 nonjoggers (those less-than-moderate exercisers) and followed them for thirty-five years. The runner/joggers exercised on average three times per week, with a weekly total of 1.1 to 2.4 hours. The results were significant: researchers noted a six to ten years increase in life expectancy for both males and female runner/joggers versus nonjoggers.

When Is More Exercise More Than Enough?

A study published in 2012, called the Aerobic Center Longitudinal Study, followed 55,137 adults for twenty-one years, comparing runners versus nonrunners. This time, these runners exercised at a more vigorous average of six miles per hour, one to two times per week, with a total average of 51 minutes per week. Results were impressive.

The investigators observed these runners to have 30 percent less risk of mortality from all causes, and 45 percent less risk from cardiovascular mortality (the greatest benefits of exercise are always cardiovascular).

Yet these researchers saw if runners exceeded 176 minutes of exercise per week, there were no additional mortality benefits. If we simply divide that into a daily average, one could speculate that an average of 25 minutes daily at six miles per hour would be considered the maximum amount to get the most mortality benefits.

That would seem to provide an answer to our question of how much is enough to gain the most mortality benefits. (Still, that does not mean you may not gain other benefits from greater amounts of exercise, such as losing weight, feelings of well-being, etc.)

When Is Extreme Too Extreme?

Many individuals participating in and training for marathons, ultra-marathons, Iron-Man Triathlons, or long-distance cycling are getting twenty to thirty times the preferred amounts of exercise needed to achieve the most mortality benefits.

A new question now surfaces: Does long-term-endurance exercise *harm the heart?*

The answer is this: While we still are not 100 percent certain, *there have been enough studies to have experts concerned.*

Before we can elaborate on what evidence has experts concerned, let us first answer, what happens in the body during these long bouts of exercise?

In other words, what are the greater demands placed on the heart during extreme sports?

Volume and Pressure

Both the left atrium and the right ventricle have thin muscular walls. Since the left atrium has only to pump blood into the adjacent left ventricle, its walls can be thin. Similarly, the right ventricle only has to pump blood to the nearby lungs. (This is different from the left ventricle, which must pump blood out to the entire body and so has thicker, more muscular walls.)

The problem is, performing extreme endurance sports will repeatedly cause a greater volume of blood and pressure into these thin-walled cavities of the heart. Over time, that can create cell damage to these structures, causing thickening and scarring of the tissue (fibrosis), making these thin muscle walls become more rigid and less elastic. That can lead to arrhythmias and other issues affecting heart function. If this occurs in the left atrium, you get atrial fibrillation. If it occurs in the right ventricle, you have ventricular arrhythmias.

As I have seen in my own practice, these are the two more commonly seen conditions in endurance sport athletes.

Studies of Concern

There have been a number of studies that point toward these kinds of possible hazards at ultra-exercise levels.

One such study looked at forty ultra-athletes who were asymptomatic (showing no symptoms). Each of them trained more than ten hours per week.

The investigators examined baseline effects occurring right after the race and then measured again a week later. To do so, they conducted cardiac MRIs to examine heart function and to determine if there had been any scarring or fibrosis that would cause heart walls to become less elastic.

Though these athletes showed no symptoms, researchers found that the right ventricle's *ejection fraction*, which measures the percentage of blood in the right ventricle being pumped out to the lungs during each beat, was reduced immediately after exercise, causing it to be less efficient. (There was no difference in the left ventricle.)

Blood tests also found an increase in *troponin I protein levels* in the blood. These are released when there has been cell damage to heart muscle. This further indicated some cell damage to the right ventricle's tissue.

The investigators also noted that those athletes who had the longest duration of activity (an ultra-marathon rather than a marathon, for example) had the greatest worsening of the right ventricle function. So the longer the duration of the sport, the greater damage to the heart.

Similarly, there was more tissue scarring in those sports with longer durations.

A Focus on Cyclists

A 2003 study (researching a 4.7-year follow-up) examined forty-six endurance athletes with a median age of thirty-one. Eighty percent were cyclists. Interestingly, each of these athletes who were studied already had some form of ventricular arrhythmias (such as PVCs, premature ventricular contractions, a fairly common condition). Of these, thirty-six felt no symptoms of the arrhythmias, while nine did experience symptoms, yet all were continuing their sport.

They followed these athletes to examine how well the right ventricle was performing. Of the forty-six athletes, researchers found that eighteen had *major arrhythmias* during their follow-up period, and nine of them died from sudden cardiac death (cardiac arrest) during that time. It should be noted all nine that died were cyclist athletes. It has been noted that cycling is one of the sports that puts the most pressure load on the heart.

The overall finding of these studies was that participation in chronic extreme sports can cause arrhythmias, including two specific types that we now will look at ARVC and atrial fibrillation.

ARVC

Arrhythmogenic right ventricular cardiomyopathy (ARVC) is normally a genetic inheritance, typically found in Italy. It is a disorder where the right ventricle muscle becomes replaced with fat and fiber and scarring over time and increases the risk of an arrhythmia and sudden cardiac death.

Yet researchers were finding similar patterns in the cardiac MRIs of these endurance athletes. One theory is that some people may possess a low level of genetic predisposition to ARVC, and the excessive endurance sport causes this transformation in the tissue to occur quicker.

The other theory is that the sports' intensity alone can create the same condition as someone who has genetic ARVC. The chronic increased pressure in the heart damages the cells and causes this accumulation of fibrous tissue.

Atrial Fibrillation

Another common arrhythmia noted in extreme sports is atrial fibrillation. This is due to the left atrium stretching from the increased intensity of exercise, leading to this fibrillation. We discussed this at length in our earlier chapter, atrial fibrillation in athletes.

Interestingly, AFib is more frequently seen in competitive cross-country runners and cross-country skiers. In fact, one study followed cross-country skiers over a period of thirty years and found AFib occurred in 13 percent of them.

Another study looked at former professional cyclists, those now at a median age of sixty-six. Even though they had stopped competing at professional levels years earlier, 10 percent of them had AFib.

More Surprises: Extreme Sports' Effects on Plaque

As said, cardiologists generally suggest exercise to reduce cardiovascular disease. Yet there are indicators that those performing *extreme sports* end up with no less cardiovascular disease than those who do not exercise.

They found that while marathon runners did have lower levels of cholesterol and several other risk factors, they had the same *calcium score*. A calcium score is the best indicator of how much plaque burden is in your arteries, which causes plaque to develop in the artery inner lining over time.

Not the Same, But Worse

Normally, marathon running and training will lower triglycerides, reduce BMI (measurement of body fat based on height and weight), and increase HDL (the good cholesterol)—all of which should lower plaque volume.

Yet another study compared marathon runners versus nonmarathon runners (most of whom were sedentary), matching them for age, blood pressure, nonsmoker or smoker, bad cholesterol, and total cholesterol. They performed CAT scans to examine everyone's plaque volume and calcium score and discovered the marathon runners had *more* plaque volume.

So while the previously mentioned study showed these levels to be the same as nonrunners (meaning marathoners were not gaining benefits), this second study showed the plaque / calcium levels of marathoners to be *worse* than those in sedentary people.

It should be noted that this increase was independent of whether the plaque was calcified or not: *Both* levels were higher. (Plaque is initially soft but over time can become more solidified and then calcified. Calcified plaque may actually be better as it is solid. Soft plaque is more vulnerable to breaking off and blocking a vessel, causing a heart attack.)

Marathoner Mystery

So what is causing marathoners to develop more plaque than people who are sedentary?

The answer may be that putting a greater amount of blood volume and pressure on the inner lining of the arteries can damage them. It can make the arteries stickier and more prone to attracting cholesterol to insert under this lining and cause blockages, just as can occur with individuals who have high blood pressure.

Also, there are changes to the electrolyte balance and metabolic changes within our tissues and blood vessels when performing extreme exercise over a long period—that can affect the integrity and damage the inner lining of the artery. While these are suggestions and not fully proven, there are new understandings that plaque found in extreme sport athletes could be different than plaque formed due to the atherosclerosis that causes heart attack. More research will shine a clearer light on this.

There is one other factor to note. Researchers observed that many involved in marathoning are not necessarily very young people. They tend to be thirty-five and older. As with much of the population, they may have had poor diets for a long time. The truth is some marathoners have unhealthy eating habits but think their exercise regimen will compensate and they will be fine. But exercise cannot negate a bad diet.

Sobering Conclusions

Overall, most studies repeatedly have shown this U-shaped phenomenon with regards to extreme sports in which there is definite benefit to cardiovascular health to a certain degree of activity. But when it is pushed beyond that, it may be causing harm.

That is not to say *everyone* will fit this pattern. Some individuals may engage in extreme sports with no apparent negative side effects. Intensity level is just one important factor, along with genetics, environment, and lifestyle. Just as some smokers seem to suffer no ill effects into old age, some extreme athletes may do the same.

But in general, we can say that excessive extreme sports are most likely harmful to your cardiovascular health. There are numerous areas of life where something is known to be good, yet *more* is not always better. This apparently applies to levels of exercise as well.

As a cardiologist, I cannot recommend that people run marathons as I do not believe it is healthful for them. Yet I would certainly advocate they do more moderate exercise, in accordance with the recommendations based on research.

Addictive

It should be noted that some extreme sports enthusiasts push themselves beyond normal limits not because they are expecting cardiovascular benefits. In truth, many commit because of what some call exercise addiction. These activities provide other benefits, as they satisfy a sense of competition, a feeling of accomplishment, a way to reduce other stresses in life.

But participants should be aware they can still have heart disease and heart attacks. I know of numerous examples, including some well-known proponents like Jim Fixx (a marathoner who published the bestseller *The Complete Book of Running* and later died of a heart attack while running).

Again, as in many things, the best answer is moderation. I cannot tell everyone that they should stop participating in these kinds of races and workouts. What I *can* do is give you the facts and let you make your own decisions. Plus, you should maintain routine checkups with your primary care physician or cardiologist. Have a calcium score performed on your heart to see how much burden is in your arteries, have advanced lipid testing that includes CRP bloodwork that reveals any markers of inflammation produced by arterial fat buildup. Having these tests performed are important enough that I have even educated primary care physicians about ordering these tests.

What is important is that if you participate in endurance sports, do not think you are immune from a heart attack. You are taking a certain amount of risk, just as there can be with other extreme activities. Skydivers, for example, understand the obvious risks they are undertaking.

Ultramarathoners need to recognize and be educated on the hidden risks they may be assuming in their sport. They need to maintain the best diets that they can and have the appropriate medical tests performed in order to safeguard their health.

CHAPTER 14

OLDER ATHLETES

Evaluating Before Exercising

Throughout this book, my intent is not to simply give you rules regarding what actions to take for your health. I want you to understand and appreciate your heart and how it functions. That way, you will be more motivated—and able—to make wise choices.

That is certainly true of the information in this chapter, which addresses the common and relevant considerations for middle-aged people desiring to exercise. Because of the inevitable aging process, and because of our society's tendency to be sedentary, middle-aged and older athletes in particular should look into getting screened to determine what type of exercise program they should undertake.

In fact, patients in this age bracket frequently come to my office, many of whom have been sedentary for many years and now wish to exercise. This includes people of all social strata, from homemakers to blue- and white-collar workers, all the way up to CEOs. I have done comprehensive executive exams for company leaders who have worked long hours for years, become overweight, and now want to get into shape. Or people who want to finally take time off and be physical, travel somewhere, and go for long hikes or ski or swim in the ocean, like they might have done years before. Or they may have limited vacation time coming up and want to get the most out of it.

I just want to make sure they do not get *too much.*

Everybody Has a Body

We sometimes forget that our body, which may have never experienced a serious medical problem in the past, must be continually cared for, especially as we age. Believe it or not, doctors can be guilty of this too, even though they should know better than anyone!

I know of a local surgeon who had become so sedentary that he was just walking to his car after a long, stressful surgery and dropped to the ground in cardiac arrest. Luckily, other nearby physicians saw him fall, immediately began CPR, and administered a defibrillator. They rushed him into the OR and opened a blockage in one of his arteries. He was fortunate to recover, as the odds of surviving cardiac arrest (where the heart completely stops pumping blood) are poor, despite all the heroic saves you might have witnessed on television.

In fact, a dentist who was obese, diabetic, and with known heart disease became stressed over something and had an arrhythmia. His heart essentially stopped functioning. Again, he was fortunate, as his office was just fifty yards from a fire station, and the paramedics were over in mere minutes to successfully shock him out of it. So what did he do? After two weeks in the hospital, he was released and back working again.

Both of these doctors had coronary events triggered by stress, which of course affects physical health. Hopefully, it will be even more obvious to readers that sedentary people in these age brackets wanting to engage in physical exercise should be checked by a physician beforehand.

This *also* holds true for people who have already been active, perhaps walking twenty minutes every day, but who now wish to partake in more intense activities. Already being active and eating well does not guarantee a person is entirely healthy. There can still be coronary risk factors that need to be evaluated. In fact, 75 percent of sudden deaths are due to heart attacks and underlying coronary artery disease for those over the age of thirty-five.

Exercise Is Good for You if Done Right

The objective of the examinations discussed in this chapter is to determine the *right* exercise for each person. Most every individual, from young to old, would benefit from exercise. Most guidelines recommend at least 150 minutes per week of moderate-intensity exercise, such as 30 minutes a day, five days a week. That could be simply brisk walking (not slow walking / talking). Just by doing this, you can lower chances of a heart attack or stroke *by 50 percent.*

If you do *high-intensity* exercise, for instance, over six miles per hour on a treadmill, you can *also* significantly lower bad cholesterol, reduce obesity, lower high blood pressure, lessen stress, diminish likelihood of arrhythmias if your body is prone to them, and improve physical fitness so your body eventually does not have to work as hard to perform the same intensity of exercise. For instance, someone who is fit could walk 20 minutes on the treadmill at three miles per hour and their heart rate only rises from 60 to 100 beats per minute, while the heart rate of someone less fit would increase from 60 to 125 for the same activity.

Again, the *highest risk* of sudden death from exercise is for those people with a sedentary lifestyle, who are overweight with abdominal obesity, have borderline blood pressure, or other possibly unknown risk factors. If they all of a sudden want to perform high-intensity activities such as skiing, singles tennis, swimming, soccer, basketball (perhaps with their kids), as if they are young again, they are dramatically increasing their chances for a heart attack.

How much an increase? The risk for someone I just described with underlying coronary disease (such as 60 to 80 percent artery blockage) who jumps into high-intensity exercise goes up *by fifty times.*

Having an exam to see what kind of exercise is appropriate, and at what intensity, *is hugely important.*

Anatomy of a Heart Attack

To better understand this, it will help to look at the mechanism behind a heart attack.

The risk is not limited only to a heart attack caused by a *sudden closure* (blockage) of an artery that cuts off blood supply to a portion of the heart muscle. With high-intensity exercise, the increased demands on the heart causes it to require more oxygen and nutrients to function. So even where there is not 100 percent closure, blood flow can still be sufficiently diminished by blockages such that there is inadequate blood supply. This can destabilize those heart's cells not getting enough oxygen and cause arrhythmias. In that case, the arrhythmias can kill you.

As said, this possibility increases during the heightened need for oxygen and nutrients during exercise. If you were not exercising, the heart continues to function and the individual has no idea there are any blockages.

If it is a *slow closure* of an artery, other blood vessels will try to compensate with more blood flow to keep delivering nourishment to the heart. But even this valiant effort by the body may not be enough to offset the increased demands placed on the heart from exercise.

Other Risks Too

To better appreciate the potential risks of exercise, it helps to know that additional changes occur in your body during exercise beyond the increased demands on the heart:

- The platelets—those blood cells that assist with clotting become stickier with exercise. This can tend to plug up arteries.
- Exercise can also cause arteries to *vasoconstrict* (narrow due to contraction of the muscular wall of the vessels), in order to *raise blood pressure* to help extremities receive increased blood flow.

Higher Altitude = Higher Risks

If one is older, exercise concerns magnify if you travel to high-altitude locations. Commonly, people visiting higher elevations are planning to ski or hike, which can be strenuous activities. While this book includes an entire chapter regarding environmental effects on athletes, let me sum up some of the information here, as it is pertinent.

There are multiple reasons to be extra cautious at elevated altitudes:

- There is lower saturation of oxygen at higher elevations, which increases the heart's workload and raises blood pressure.
- The dehydration naturally experienced at high altitudes worsens the situation. If you develop an electrolyte imbalance, such as from increased perspiration from exercise, you further amplify the risk.
- Travel by airplane can add to further dehydration, as airplane air is quite dry.
- Do not believe the myth that your body can acclimate to higher altitudes within just one or two days. For what we are discussing here, the body requires more time to adjust. How long that takes will at least partially depend on the altitude to which you are traveling.
- It should be noted here again that if you take a stimulant, such as caffeine, before exercise, you additionally raise blood pressure and risk.

Does this mean all people must refrain from exercising when traveling to higher altitudes?

It largely comes down to how active you have been beforehand. If you are very fit and run a few miles daily with no symptoms, you should be able to continue the same exercise (though at lower intensity). You still need to be extra conscientious to make sure you drink enough fluids (not caffeine). For those less fit, you should consult with your doctor about what levels of activity would be safe for you.

Evaluation of Sedentary Older Individuals

People over thirty-five may wonder if they need testing before they begin an activity or exercise. The answer depends on the intensity of the proposed activity and the person's health.

Doctors can define intensity of an exercise by using a standard called *metabolic equivalent* or *metabolic expenditure* (MET).

- A person simply sitting and doing nothing else is expending an energy of one MET.
- Any activity between one and three METs is considered low-intensity exercise (such as normal walking).
- Between three and six METs is considered moderate intensity (brisk walking from three to six miles per hour, or doubles tennis).
- Anything over six METs is considered high-intensity exercise (skiing, cycling, singles tennis, swimming).

If a sedentary individual with no symptoms and no other risk factors (no hypertension or diabetes) wants to do low-intensity exercise—less than three METs of exercise (gentle walking)—they do not need to do any tests. They can start walking slowly.

If a sedentary person wants to begin moderate exercise—between three and six METs—they should do a treadmill stress test.

If someone sedentary wants to participate in high-intensity exercise, they should certainly do a stress test, but we do not recommend that a sedentary individual dive into high-intensity activities.

Determining Health Status of Sedentary Individuals

Doctors also factor in the person's health in deciding what testing should be performed and what activities will be safe.

So how do we determine a *sedentary person's* level of health?

First, we have you complete the Physical Activity Readiness Questionnaire (PARQ). Questions include whether you have high blood pressure, symptoms of chest pain or shortness of breath, symptoms of dizziness or light-headedness or feel you might pass out, or if a doctor has ever previously said that you need to limit your exercise.

Even when your plan is only to do low-intensity exercise, if you respond yes to even one of these queries, then stress testing must be done before you can be cleared for exercise. If the stress test is normal, you can move forward with the exercise.

On the other hand, a middle-aged person that is physically active, physically fit, and with no symptoms who wants to do low-intensity exercise of zero to three METs may participate without testing or completing the questionnaire.

But if they want to do moderate exercise—three to six METs— they should complete the PARQ. If any of their answers are positive, they should also have further testing. But if all answers are negative and there are no symptoms, they can participate in the physical activity without a stress test.

If they want to do high-intensity exercise—over six METs— then in addition to completing the questionnaire, they should be seen by a doctor (preferably a cardiologist) and have a full workup. This includes the following:

+ Personal and family history
+ A physical
+ Calculated risk score
+ A baseline EKG

Based on those results, the doctor can decide if a stress test is advisable.

Frequency of Reevaluations

Obviously, our bodies are always changing. We age, our diet varies, our exercise regimen may alter or be inconsistent, so once you are tested and given a green light to exercise, when should you be *retested*?

If you experience any symptoms, you should be retested.

If no symptoms, you should be reevaluated at least once a year. That may not mean performing another stress test. But it does include your completing the questionnaire again and getting a physical from a doctor as well as reviewing your physical history.

Self-Evaluate?

Patients who wish to get some sense of their own heart health can use a self-diagnostic tool, such as the Framingham Risk Score. Available on my website under the Resources page, it is an algorithm that asks a number of questions, including your age and your lab test results, and estimates the risk percentage of your having a cardiac event in the next ten years.

While this valuable tool can help a patient *recognize if they are at greater risk*, it is not the whole picture.

Do not simply fill out the questionnaire and think (especially if you are sedentary) that a good score indicates you are low risk. It is not that simple. For instance, a sedentary person's result might show the risk of having a heart attack within the next ten years as 10 percent. Someone physically active but who has some medical history could get the same risk score. But the reality is the sedentary person has a much higher chance of heart attack than the one who is physically active. In fact, a study showed that a middle-aged thin or lean woman who is sedentary has a much higher risk of having a heart attack than an obese woman who exercises regularly.

What I am saying is you should not merely self-diagnose. A doctor's expertise is required to truly understand your heart's health.

Guidelines

Cardiologists in the United States follow a couple of different guidelines to determine when patients should be tested before exercising. One is from the American Heart Association, while the other is from European Society of Cardiology.

The American Heart Association (AHA) says that all men over the age of forty and all females over the age of fifty should have a further workup before they do any exercise if they have any one of the following:

- Family history of parents with coronary disease—heart attack, stroke, bypass, stent, angioplasty—if it was a male under fifty-five or female under sixty-five.
- Any symptoms at all (chest pressure, palpitations, dizziness, etc.).
- Any abnormality on their cardiovascular physical exam (heart murmur, abnormal EKG, irregular pulse, etc.).

Further, the AHA recommends that *everyone* over the age of sixty-five, even if they have zero risk factors or symptoms, should have a stress test.

Plus, as indicated previously, if a person has any symptoms or is intending to perform higher-intensity exercise, they should have a stress test on an annual basis.

Personally, even though this is not part of the official AHA guidelines, my recommendation is that someone over sixty-five do a treadmill test every year, as one can develop a new undetected blockage within that period of time.

The other recommendations we may use come from the European Society of Cardiology (ESC) Guidelines. To determine if patients need further testing, they consider three factors:

- Individual's medical risk for heart attack
- If the person is already exercising and their level of physical activity
- The type of sport intended for participation

Individual doctors in the United States might follow one or the other set of criteria, or a combination of both, in determining when more comprehensive testing should be given to patients.

Treadmill Testing Accuracy

As much as we wish it were not the case, like many tests, stress tests are not 100 percent accurate. A simple treadmill test, with no imaging done at the same time, is only 70 percent accurate in detecting tight blockages.

If you add imaging, like stress echo, the accuracy moves up to 90 percent.

It should be noted the same 90 percent accuracy occurs if you do nuclear imaging instead of stress echo. With nuclear imaging, a radioactive isotope is injected into the patient's vein during rest and after exercise. We compare the two readings to see if the radioactive isotope is taken up by the heart muscle at rest and during exercise. The patient could have a tight blockage that is not apparent when they are at rest, but during the higher demands of physical stress, the heart does not receive sufficient blood supply. In that case, less radioactive isotope will be detected in the portion of the muscle supplied by the artery.

So if testing has less than 100 percent accuracy, is it still worth doing?

A resounding yes.

It could reveal an otherwise unknown blockage and save your life.

Yet there is good news even when there is a false negative (an existing blockage is not detected). While a regular treadmill test, particularly one with no imaging, *can* result in a false negative, studies show that the risk of heart attack is much less for someone who has the false negative on their treadmill test than someone who has a true positive result.

Why is that?

If you get a false negative, you have less chance of a heart attack because the false negative likely means the blockage is of a more minor nature. For example, it might be there is a borderline one-artery blockage with 80 percent closure (as opposed to 99 percent). Plus, the individual's body may have developed collateral veins that bring enough blood to the heart to supply sufficient nourishment.

But if another person does the stress test and there is a significant abnormality (positive result), then they are clearly at a higher risk of sudden death from a heart attack.

Bottom Line: Do Not Assume

Hopefully it is clear that even if you have not experienced any symptoms of heart disease, it is critically important to be evaluated before commencing an exercise program. This is especially true for people over thirty-five. Yes, going to see the doctor and getting tested can be a hassle, but it is *so much less* of a burden than having a heart attack and possibly dying or surviving but with chances of a lifelong weakened heart.

Take care of yourself and your body.

It is the only one you get!

SPECIAL CIRCUMSTANCES

For Athletes

CHAPTER 15

ENVIRONMENT AND ATHLETIC PERFORMANCE

We have discussed how athletic performance and well-being is dramatically affected by our health, fitness level, diet, age, etc.

Yet there is another factor we should discuss.

We do not live in isolation. We live in the world, and the environmental conditions of that world can affect our performance and our health in important ways you may not have considered.

Exercising in a Hot Environment

Body temperature is critical to our health, especially during exercise. Our core temperature needs to remain within a narrow range for our body to perform well and for us to stay alive. Obviously the ambient (outside) temperature can play a factor. But we must also keep in mind that any physical activity puts extra demands on our body and its ability to maintain a proper core temperature. Exercise warms our body since muscle contractions generate heat.

Exercising in hot temperatures can pose challenges to our body. High humidity levels can further magnify these effects.

I frequently cite that our body is remarkable. This is true again in its efforts to maintain our core temperature within the required limits. If our core temperature rises too much, the body attempts to cool itself off.

So how does our body avoid becoming too warm?

The body compensates by increasing blood flow to the skin, which generates sweat from the sweat glands. This sweat on your skin then evaporates to cool your body.

This is why it is so important to keep hydrated, as we must have sufficient fluid in our system in order to sweat. If we are dehydrated, our body is unable to produce this needed perspiration. The result is less sweat evaporation and reduced cooling. This can contribute to *hyperthermia*, excessive heat in the body.

In addition to being integral for thermal regulation, water enables better athletic performance in other ways as well. If your body has inadequate fluid, it can negatively affect the cardiac output and amount of blood that can be circulated to vital organs. Such dehydration can cause kidney damage if there is not enough blood flow to the kidney.

How Much Water Is Enough?

If you are an athlete, you must look at three factors to determine how much you should be drinking: thirst, urine, weight.

- If you are thirsty, your body is indicating that you are dehydrated.
- If your urine color is dark yellow, this indicates dehydration.
- If your weight is lower than normal, it may also signify you are not drinking enough fluids.

An athlete, or anyone for that matter, should look at these variables every day. Some athletes try to address this issue by drinking an abundance of *only* water. But if you drink too much water, it can lead to *hyponatremia*, a condition where the sodium level in your blood is abnormally low, since the surplus water is diluting the sodium concentration.

Sodium is an electrolyte that helps regulate how much water there is in and around your cells. If the amount of sodium is insufficient, your cells can begin to swell. Symptoms can include confusion, nausea, vomiting, diminished energy or fatigue, seizures, and unconsciousness. This swelling can be mild to life-threatening.

Compounding this issue is that if you sweat a lot, you also lose additional salt (sodium). That is why it is important when exercising not to simply hydrate with water but to also drink something like Gatorade that contains electrolytes (including sodium). Or eat salty foods containing sufficient sodium to compensate for the loss.

Muscle Cramps

If you are dehydrated and/or exercise in a hot environment, you can develop mild to severe symptoms.

The mildest of these is when electrolyte imbalances in your muscles affect how the muscle contracts and functions. This leads to cramps. In these circumstances, your core temperature may be elevated, but still less than 104 degrees Fahrenheit. The basic treatment for this is fluid intake accompanied by salt to replenish your sodium level. Water alone is not enough. You need to consume water and salt, or just Gatorade.

Passing Out from Heat Syncope

More serious symptoms can occur in someone who is not an athlete and has been sedentary. If they exercise in a hot environment, they can pass out due to something called *venous pooling*. Excess blood accumulates (pools) in the veins of their legs and cannot sufficiently pump back to the heart. This occurs because the person is not used to exercise, and the veins in their legs have not adapted to being more efficient under the stress of exercise. As less blood volume travels to the heart, less blood is then pumped to the brain, and the person can lose consciousness. This is called *heat syncope*.

Someone suffering from heat syncope will have pulse and respiratory rates that are not excessively high (unlike when you are dehydrated and the heart rate increases to compensate). While the body's core temperature can be elevated, it is still less than 104 degrees.

If we try to immediately assess such a patient, and note that pulse, respiratory rates, and temperature are all normal, we can likely determine they passed out due to heat syncope, since these variables are not at the higher levels associated with other conditions. While temperature may be *slightly* elevated, the athlete may exhibit dizziness, light-headedness, pale or weary skin, tunnel vision, or weakness.

Heat Exhaustion

A potentially more serious condition, *heat exhaustion* usually includes such symptoms as confusion, nausea, vomiting, and severe tiredness in response to exercise. The person's temperature is elevated but still less than 104. But in this case, their heart rate is elevated (over one hundred beats per minute).

Heat exhaustion can also lead to heat stroke. The person should rest in a cool, shady spot or sit in front of a fan. Getting the athlete into an air-conditioned building is best. Drink cool fluids (water only).

Heat Stroke

The most severe condition, *heat stroke*, can cause someone to end up in the emergency room and very possibly die. Heat stroke occurs when the body temperature climbs over 104. It is accompanied with severe mental disorientation (confusion), nausea, and vomiting. The human body simply cannot tolerate such a high inner core temperature.

If they can be diagnosed as experiencing heat stroke (body temperature over 104, telltale symptoms of confusion, nausea and vomiting), this person must be *immediately prevented* from further exercise or activity. Call 911 while you try to cool their body as fast as possible. This can be done by pouring ice water over them, if available. Yet even if they start to feel better, they need to go to the ER right away and be placed in an ice water bath.

People are at higher risk of heat stroke if they are obese and not physically fit.

Coaches Do Not Always Know

Athletes can experience heatstroke too. I usually hear of this happening to overweight linemen trying out for a football team. During the first few weeks, coaches are weeding out players by requiring very rigorous exercises. These practices are often where we get the news stories of young athletes dying from heat stroke. Plus, these young men are already wearing heavy clothes and gear. Their bodies cannot sweat to cool off.

Coaches who are not educated continually push these young men. If the athlete begins to fatigue, the coach pushes them harder! Even if the coach does possess the knowledge, *the athlete* should understand these risks to their health and *protect themselves*. The athlete must be their own best advocate and not assume the coach always knows best. A life may hang in the balance.

Fortunately, from my place in the world of soccer, I can attest to the progress that has been made in educating coaches. Coaches have to renew their credentials every two years, which includes learning about the risks of heat stroke, concussions, etc.

A person can be at higher risk of heat stroke if they are on certain medications, especially ephedrine types like Akovaz and Corphedra (different names for the same drug) or methylphenidate drugs for ADHD. People being treated for ADHD must be especially careful regarding heat stroke. That is because drugs used to treat ADHD contain ephedrine-type ingredients, which can potentially lead to heat stroke.

Exercising in a Cold Environment

At the other end of the temperature spectrum is physical activity in a cold setting.

Hypothermia

When the body is exposed to cold air, the skin receptors send signals to the sympathetic nervous system. That causes narrowing (vasoconstriction) of the arterial vessels so there is less heat loss. The nose, fingers, and cheeks are particularly sensitive to this vasoconstriction, and that can lead to frostbite. Also, the body's temperature regulator, the hypothalamus, sends signals to the muscles to shiver to generate heat to warm the body.

Hypothermia occurs when your core body temperature drops below 95 degrees Fahrenheit. This results when heat loss occurs faster than your body can compensate by generating its own heat.

Here are five stages to hypothermia (with the likely Fahrenheit temperature range in which they occur):

+ Mild—shivering with normal (or near normal) consciousness (32–35 degrees)
+ Moderate—shivering ceases but consciousness is impaired (28–32 degrees)
+ Severe—approaching death (24–28 degrees)
+ Apparent Death—extremely close to death (15–24 degrees)
+ Death from irreversible hypothermia

Treatment for Serious Hypothermia

Obviously, call 911 if you can. Cover the person with layers of dry coats or blankets, including their head (though not their face). Protect them against wind and cold, but do not massage or rub the skin to warm them up. Avoid strenuous or jolting motions as that could provoke a cardiac arrest. Try to insulate them with coats from the cold ground (it conducts more heat from the body). If possible, take them indoors to a warm environment. Gently remove any wet clothing. If needed (and possible), you may cut away these wet clothes to prevent unnecessary motion. Try to keep the person in a horizontal position.

Continually check their condition, realizing that someone with severe hypothermia may seem to be unconscious, without obvious breathing or even a pulse. If their breathing is perilously shallow or nonexistent, perform CPR if you are trained.

To keep them warm, you can give warm beverages (not alcoholic or caffeinated) if they can swallow. Do not apply a hot water bottle or heating pad. Such direct heat can injure the skin or even trigger irregular rhythms that can lead to cardiac arrest.

There are other steps you can take as well. If you know you are venturing into a cold environment, it is best that you read about first-aid procedures ahead of time for someone suffering from hypothermia.

One group of people more susceptible to hypothermia are those individuals with less body fat, since fat acts as an insulator that can help the body retain warmth.

Another group at greater risk for hypothermia during exercise are those over sixty. This is because as we get older, our vasculature, hormonal system, brain, and neurological musculoskeletal system all function less efficiently. Plus, people over sixty tend to be at higher risk for underlying cardiovascular disease.

Aging Process: a Personal Story

Our bodies function and recover less effectively as we age. I know this personally (even though I am under sixty), and I have been an athlete all my life.

I had a knee injury some years ago that limited me tremendously for eighteen months. Years before this, I could easily play soccer with the kids that I coached. But because of my year and a half of little exercise due to my injury, even as my knee was feeling better, I could barely walk faster than a normal pace.

During this time, I was in Germany getting advanced training to perform transcatheter aortic valve replacement (TAVR), a leading-edge technology that cardiologists were just beginning to perform. Much less invasive than open-heart surgery, the cardiologist accesses the body through an artery in the leg to put a new valve into the heart. Recovery time, patient longevity, and a lowered risk of stroke are all the benefits to this technique that make it superior to open-heart surgery. Patients can go home the next day!

I was thrilled to be there to learn this new technique. Yet when I walked even the short distance to the hospital from the hotel in cold weather, I would experience dizziness and tachycardia (a heart rate over one hundred beats per minute).

During the time I had been injured, I had gained some weight, and my body had decompensated significantly. I could no longer handle even a little physical or mental stress. I would get palpitations, dizziness, light-headedness such that I would have to sit down.

Slowly as my knee improved, I began exercising. First ten minutes, then fifteen, twenty, then thirty minutes. I increased my speed as well. Now I routinely do thirty minutes of treadmill daily, along with a few days of rowing per week. By exercising, my body and mind now compensate well again, even with the mental stress that accompanies my profession.

Your Personal Environment: Clothing

Another factor that can lead to a greater chance of hypothermia in cold weather is wet clothing. To keep clothing from becoming saturated with sweat (wet), it is recommended that anyone exercising in a cold environment wear *three layers* of clothes. The two inner layers should be polyester. These are superior to cotton as they wick moisture away from the body. The outer layer should be some type of thin rain gear that prevents the inner layers from becoming wet due to inclement weather and also keeps out the wind. Wind, rain, and cold can dramatically lower your body core temperature. However, if it is not rainy or windy, skip the outer rain gear / windbreaker and just wear the two inner layers.

Of course, if your environment is particularly cold and you need more warmth, you can wear an additional layer (of polyester). If it is *still* too cold, you might skip going outside that day and find a way to exercise indoors.

As you exercise and your body warms up, you can remove some of these layers. That is why, in part, it is recommended to wear three layers. You not only control susceptibility to wind and rain, you can also better regulate body temperature.

Frostbite

Besides hypothermia, there are a couple of other conditions that can occur in a cold environment that are dangerous.

The worst of these is frostbite. This occurs when cold outside temperatures result in a lack of oxygen to the body tissues. This is due to *vasospasm*, a constriction of blood capillaries (tiny vessels) in response to the freezing cold. This causes a reduction of blood flow. The affected tissue does not get sufficient oxygen nourishment from the blood. Symptomatically, the tissue first shows edema (accumulation of fluid in tissues or circulatory system) and swelling. Subsequently, the tissue turns blue (cyanotic) because of insufficient blood flow.

We are susceptible to frostbite when tissue is exposed to cold wet temperatures below thirty-two degrees Fahrenheit or zero degrees centigrade for long periods of time (hours, not minutes). It typically affects the most exposed areas first: nose, ears, fingers, and toes. There is no immediate sensation of pain, yet it results in tissue damage and, in more extreme cases, may require amputation of the dead body tissues.

Frostbite will occur when the temperature *of the body tissue* goes below seventy degrees Fahrenheit. Do not confuse this number with outside temperature figures. Body tissues typically maintain a normal temperature even when ambient temperatures are cold. But if outside conditions are cold enough, the body tissue is unable to maintain healthy levels.

Obviously, you cannot measure when body tissues go below seventy degrees, but you can use the following information as a guide to know when you are at greater risk:

- Frostbite risks increase significantly when windy with a low outside temperature.
- Frostbite will not occur if air temperature is more than thirty-two degrees Fahrenheit.
- But that number must take into account *the wind-chill factor*.

How can you estimate the wind-chill factor? A good approximation is to multiply the wind speed by 0.7 and subtract that number from actual air temperature.

For example, it is thirty-five degrees Fahrenheit outside with a wind speed of ten miles per hour.

- First multiply 10 x 0.7 = 7
- Then do the subtraction 35 − 7 = 28

You would have an equivalent temperature of twenty-eight degrees Fahrenheit.

You can begin to see how when you have strong winds, coupled with colder temperatures, that the effective temperature (including wind-chill) really goes down.

It should be noted there is a second way that one can develop frostbite too: by touching very cold metal. Metal is a very good conductor of cold and can cause frostbite to develop quite quickly.

Tissue Damage in Less Cold Temperatures Is Possible Too

Tissue injuries can also occur when exercising in less than extreme cold temperatures, which can be called *non-freezing cold injuries.*

Trench foot is just such an example. It describes when there are wet conditions within one's socks, in cold temperatures (though not freezing cold), for long periods of time. The wet cold causes constriction of the blood vessels, leading to insufficient blood flow to the feet. This can first result in numbness of the feet, which then turn blue (indicating lack of oxygen). There may be pain, with this leading to deterioration of tissue in the feet. This too can cause damage, even though it is not actually frostbite.

You can best avoid this condition through keeping your feet dry by changing socks several times during extended exercise. Also, keeping active in such conditions helps keep the feet warm. In other words, do not exercise such that your feet become wet and cold and then decide to walk or stand still for long periods. Onset can be as rapid as ten hours of cold wet conditions.

High Altitudes

Moving our focus away from ambient temperatures, I am now going to address altitude. While weather conditions typically will be colder at higher elevations, my attention is on the amount of oxygen at different altitudes and their effects on athletes.

As you gain elevation, there is a smaller percentage of oxygen in the air. You may be breathing the same volume of air, but your tissues are receiving less oxygen. The body tries to compensate by increasing your breathing rate and increasing your cardiac output (which circulates oxygen-carrying blood) by raising your heart rate.

Because of this, when athletes train or compete at higher altitudes, the body will become stressed and tire more quickly than usual. You would be well advised to take more time and more breaks to complete the same task. Fortunately, in most cases, your body can acclimate and recover 90 percent of its efficiency after spending a week's time at this altitude.

Low, Moderate, High, and Very High Altitudes

Let us first understand what is meant by the various descriptions of altitude:

- Low altitude is less than 1,200 meters, or 3,937 feet.
- Moderate altitude is between 1,200 to 2,400 meters, or 3,937 to 7,874 feet.
- High altitude (where problems start) is over 2,400 meters, which is 7,874 feet.
- Very high altitude is over 4,000 meters, meaning over 13,123 feet.

When your body cannot compensate for the diminished oxygen, you may experience various medical situations.

Acute Mountain Sickness

Acute mountain sickness (AMS) is the least severe reaction. It usually happens when you travel up the mountain to a high level very rapidly (rapid ascent). This could be driving to a high altitude, such as ten thousand feet, to go skiing. The main symptoms can include headache, nausea, fatigue, and inability to speak clearly.

Whether you experience this depends on the altitude and your physical condition, as well as various other body factors. But in general:

- At moderate altitudes, this condition occurs to 15 percent of people.
- At high altitudes, this happens 15 to 70 percent of people.
- At very high altitudes, this takes place with over 70 percent of people.

As soon as you notice these symptoms, in yourself or in someone with you, immediately stop whatever activity you are engaged in. Then either stay at that altitude (do not go any higher) or go down to lower altitudes. Symptoms usually disappear within forty-eight hours.

High-Altitude Cerebral Edema

If you are having acute mountain sickness and you do not stop activity or you keep ascending to higher altitudes, you may experience the more serious condition of *high-altitude cerebral edema* (HACE). This is swelling of the brain. Symptoms are similar to acute mountain sickness, but much more extreme. It is best to recognize the condition as soon as possible, particularly if you are alone, since as the condition worsens, the person becomes unable to descend on their own.

With HACE, it is recommended to descend one thousand to three thousand feet and sleep. If available, supplemental oxygen or even time in a hyperbaric (decompression) chamber can aid recovery.

These conditions, and suggested treatment, can apply to anyone at elevated altitudes. But if you are exerting, through strenuous sports (skiing, running) or by carrying extra weight (backpacking/climbing), your chances are greater to suffer one of these conditions.

High-Altitude Pulmonary Edema

An even more severe condition is *high-altitude pulmonary edema* (HAPE). This means fluid has entered your lungs. This is a very serious situation because it indicates your heart is functioning inadequately, your tissues are getting insufficient oxygen, and though your body is trying to compensate, your condition has degraded beyond what the body can counter.

The reduced oxygen and pressure in the ambient air is affecting the air pressure within the lungs, causing fluid to leave the tissues to enter the lungs. Once fluid is in the lungs, less air can come in to oxygenate the blood, and your condition worsens. This carries a high risk for mortality. This occurs more often if you go very high very fast, then go down fast, and then up fast again. An example of such an activity could be downhill skiing. Early symptoms of this condition would be sore throat and coughing. These alone may not be interpreted as serious by the typical lay person, but they are possible indicators of the much more acute underlying condition.

So pay attention if these develop in you or someone with you!

Essentially, when at altitude, *pay attention to any symptoms.* Do not consider them minor inconveniences to be ignored or powered through. They may be the body's warning of potentially life-threating conditions. If you see them in someone with you, do not let that person brush off your concerns. That could cost them their life! It is *your* time to be responsible for *them*.

Acclimation

Symptoms occur when the body has to suddenly compensate for a dramatic increase in altitude and reduction in oxygen. This is why it is best to go up a mountain very slowly. After remaining at a high altitude for a week, the body can physiologically compensate to the stressors and lack of oxygen.

Again, the body is incredible. One way it adapts is by increasing red blood cell production from the bone marrow. Even though you are still taking in less oxygen, the increase in red blood cells can better deliver that oxygen to the tissues.

Some people have a misconception that they can acclimate in a much shorter time. They might drive up to a high altitude, rest overnight or a couple of nights, and think they are good to go for some strenuous hike or skiing. Depending on their age, physical condition, and the altitude, they might get away with it. Or they might not. But even if they do not get symptoms on this occasion, that may not be true next time. Perhaps the altitude will be higher, the activity level greater, your body is not in as good of shape as it was the first time, or you are older.

This is not about mental attitude. Sudden increases in elevation will *affect every body*. That needs to be understood and respected. You cannot push through it or tough it out. Do not let others provoke you to do something that you know is a bad idea.

This is science. It is not about your attitude. It is about *altitude*.

Environmental Conditions Need Not Be Extreme

One does not have to be high on a mountain or in blizzard conditions for the body to experience ill effects due to environmental exposures. While the scenarios given so far point to more intense climatic conditions, one should always be conscious of what may be occurring outside *and inside* their body.

Let me share a firsthand report as example.

Cold outside temperatures cause constriction of the arteries (to maintain heat within the body), which makes the heart work harder to pump against the greater restrictions. This happened a few weeks ago to someone I know who was coaching soccer at night when it was very cold. Though only wearing a short-sleeve shirt with a light jacket and shorts, he was actively moving up and down the field.

Yet after one hour, he began feeling poorly. He had access to a blood pressure device, and knowing he already had borderline high blood pressure, he measured his to discover it was at 170. He knew enough to go home and warm himself up for a few hours beneath a blanket until he felt better and his blood pressure dropped to his normal range. He ultimately was fine.

Caught up in the game, he was not feeling cold even when temperatures cooled off as the night progressed because his body was compensating by constricting blood vessels. But even though the level of activity (running up and down the sidelines) was not that intense, he began feeling like he was overexerting.

I tell this story because there can be times when we do not pay adequate heed to our environment, and even if we start to feel something is off, we may tell ourselves that we can tough it out. But *our body response* cannot be countered by adopting an "I'm tough as nails" attitude.

It is this same automatic body response that makes shoveling snow in the winter dangerous for many people who are older and/or have borderline high blood pressure. (The same can be true for swimming in waters that are too cold.)

Such concerns are greater at the beginning of your activity as the body does warm up as you exercise. That is why we advise you to start your activity by wearing layers that you can remove, or at least unzip, as you exercise. However, when shoveling snow, depending on how aggressively you shovel, your body may not warm up sufficiently to offset its typical blood vessel constricting to keep you warm. Therein lies the danger behind the warnings that physicians voice every snow season.

The same can still hold true if exercising in extreme cold. Your body warming up from movement may not be sufficient to counteract intense outdoor temperatures.

In less than extreme conditions, these concerns are most applicable to those who are older or already have blood pressure or other heart issues. The body of a young healthy person without blood pressure issues could compensate to handle this situation (as did the young soccer players at that game).

The bottom line is, again, be knowledgeable, be aware, and pay attention.

CHAPTER 16

MISUSE OF PERFORMANCE-ENHANCING DRUGS BY ATHLETES

In the United States, there is great pressure to function at our maximum potential. It is touted as a highly laudable aspiration within our culture. Books, seminars, and high-priced keynote speeches all promise to motivate and educate toward this end. To give us that "edge."

Nearly no arena pushes limits more than athletic competition does.

No longer are sports viewed primarily as a means to build character, where sometimes you win and sometimes you lose: When you win, you are grateful. When you lose, you learn from your mistakes and come back stronger to compete again. A formula for improving performance *and* building character.

This is the approach we *should* have.

But the prevailing attitude today is that *winning is everything.* With victory comes attention, accolades, and admirers. For a professional athlete, compensations can include enhanced salary, plus financial endorsements from companies and organizations.

All this spurs many athletes to win at any cost. Sometimes that includes turning to performance-enhancing drugs to give them that edge. To become superhuman (almost).

Medications Misused

All medications exist to counter a physical ailment. Even so, and as positive as medications can be, they all come with some risk. As physicians, we always weigh any risk against potential benefits before we recommend any drug to a patient.

The athletic community and some sketchy companies with dark labs that cater to it have found ways to use some drugs intended for legitimate medical purposes (sometimes enhancing components of a drug's action) to improve athletic performance. Neither they nor the athletes are considering long-term side effects. But only short-term immediate results.

Many of these products go far beyond those improve-your-performance supplements that one can find in athletic magazine ads. These are essentially illegal drugs that athletes (and sometimes their coaches) acquire under the radar.

This can include nonprofessional level players as well.

Starts Young

With my own eyes, I saw the coach of an opposing team of highly competitive youth soccer players give every one of his players a pill. These were thirteen-to-fifteen-year-olds! I do not know what those pills contained, but whatever it was, I am confident it wasn't legal.

Coaches of youth teams are supposed to protect their young players and serve as role models. But because of social (*and parental*) emphasis on winning, some coaches take it too far. This goes beyond passing out pills. Coaches drive these kids to triumph at all costs, which can stress out children and promote unhealthy risk-taking.

Parents need to know that this happens. And that they may be partly responsible as they crave success for their kid's team. All this can have lasting and negative effects on their kids. As the saying goes, winning isn't everything. (And no, it's *not* "the only thing.")

Coaches wield a great deal of influence. Both nonprofessional and professional athletes believe that whatever the coach says goes.

But coaches have their own agendas.

At college and professional levels, coaches are lured by the money and fame that comes along with having a successful team. Yet such an imbalance exists even with youth teams. A winning year gives that coach prestige and bragging rights and brings better players to their team the following season. In fact, some youth teams, such as those in the East Bay (Silicon Valley) of San Francisco, use professional coaches. British-accented individuals with various licenses who are paid by the parents. It is conceivable that parents of any player accepted to one of these elite teams will pay between six to ten thousand dollars a year to the league, which then gives some of that money to the coaches, conditioned in part on a winning record.

The attitudes toward youth sports as reflected in these examples need to change. Our children would be far better served if we go back to where competition is not *only* about winning. The glory of winning *and* the heartbreak of losing both build character, which should be the main goal of having our youth participate in sports.

In addition to that, young people learning about teamwork bestows benefits on them for the rest of their life. A study was conducted to find out the single most important factor in "creating" the best surgeons in the United States. Turns out, it was not the schools they attended. It was not the medical board scores they attained. The most consistent single element was whether they played a team sport in college. It is the team that helps you score a goal, sink a basket, run the bases, or save a life.

This applies not just to doctors but also to many careers and aspects of life.

Let us take a look at the most frequently abused types of medications.

Anabolic Steroids

One of the most commonly misused drugs is anabolic steroids.

There are legitimate medical uses for these steroids, as in the treatment of delayed puberty, people with muscle wasting, and for some men, experiencing impotence. Anabolic steroid hormones are naturally produced in your body, the main one being testosterone.

While medical use for testosterone replacement is meant only to reproduce normal hormone levels in the blood, testosterone used illegally by some athletes can be in far higher doses (as well as combined with other chemical substances to increase muscle-building).

Side effects of testosterone supplementation in men can include the following:

+ Acne
+ Development of breast tissue like females
+ Small testicles

While some readers expect testosterone supplementation might *increase* testicle size, a little medical knowledge makes it very obvious why the opposite is true. Testicles make testosterone. If you provide that steroid through supplementation, the testicles no longer have to make it. So they atrophy.

For women, testosterone supplementation can cause the following:

+ Enlarged Adam's apple
+ Excessive body hair

Further, if young people use anabolic steroids, it can prematurely close the plates on bones, leading to stunted growth. Such a person will not reach a normal range of height or weight. Aside from the potential lifelong harm to self-esteem, this can also lead to long-term health issues. Further, such testosterone supplementation can affect those parts of the brain called the amygdala or hypothalamus, causing aggressive behavior that can lead to a fracturing of relationships, as well as physical harm to others or oneself.

There is an additional problem as well: If you have been taking testosterone and recognize you are being negatively affected and suddenly stop taking it, it can cause you to experience acute withdrawal that can lead to depression and even suicide.

Another class of anabolic steroids is called SARM (selective androgen receptor modulator). Versions of this, named Ostarine or LGD-4033, are illegally made by dark labs for use by athletes. Hormone modulators such as these are not FDA approved for *any* human use or consumption. These types of drugs can cause toxicity in the liver, as well as lower your HDL (good cholesterol), leading to atherosclerosis (plaque formation in arteries), premature heart attacks, and strokes. Heart attacks and strokes are thought of issues that come with aging. Yet these can manifest in young people due to SARM supplementation.

Corticosteroids

Other steroids called *corticosteroids* lower inflammation in the body and are used to treat allergies, allergic reactions, and diseases like asthma. Examples of these are Prednisolone and Solu Medrol. Athletes abuse these drugs as they can give a lot of fast energy when you first use it. Of course, there can be serious side effects as well, including growth retardation, diabetes, anxiety, and tremors.

Peptide Hormones

This class of hormones includes growth hormones, erythropoietin, and adrenocorticotropic hormone (ACTH).

Growth hormones are produced in the body by the pituitary gland in the brain. Some people like to supplement with this as it can increase lean body mass (muscle) while lowering fatty mass. This is particularly appealing to swimmers. While not a steroid, it *is* anabolic, which means it stimulates growth, as it improves carbohydrate and fat metabolism.

Normally, females have higher levels of growth hormones than males, peaking during puberty. After that, for every ten years, growth hormone production decreases by 14 percent for both sexes.

Yet if you want to increase the amount of growth hormone in your body, you can do so *naturally*—with exercise. Prolonged moderate exercise of over an hour (an example being 3 to 4.6 mph on a steep treadmill) *can increase release of growth hormone from your pituitary gland by ten times.* Alternatively, if you do just ten to twenty minutes of intense exercise (running, soccer, or swimming), you can still boost release of natural growth hormone by five to ten times.

People generally think exercise helps them lose weight and build leaner bodies because of calories expended and thus become discouraged when they learn an hour of exercise burns only 150 calories, which can equal just one chocolate bar. Some people then think, "So why bother?"

Why bother?

Because there are all kinds of other benefits that go far beyond just expending calories, many of which are described elsewhere in this book. I mention again the increased release of growth hormone, an increase in metabolism that gives you benefits all day, improved sleep, chemical release that improves mood, control of insulin / blood sugar levels, strengthening of bones, diminishing some cancer risks, and lessening chances of heart disease.

The higher the intensity of exercise, the more growth hormones released.

Getting the Right Amounts of Human Growth Hormone

While you may wish to *increase* the amount of human growth hormones (HGH) in your body, you need to know certain conditions or actions *reduce* amounts of human growth hormones.

Eating lots of carbohydrate-rich foods lowers the amounts of growth hormone. But if you do not overeat and eat only when hungry and in small portions, you benefit from a greater release of growth hormone.

It is important to also know that obesity lowers release of growth hormone. This is unfortunate, as another positive aspect of growth hormone is that it causes lipolysis, which breaks down fat from the abdomen and redistributes it to areas outside the central part of your body. That is important, as central obesity has been proven to be dangerous for risk of diabetes and heart attacks.

At the same time, *too much* growth hormone increases retention of fluids in your body, which can lead to hypertension.

That is why HGH supplements must be used correctly (if at all) to be truly beneficial. If taking one to two international units (IU) per day, you can get a lot of the benefits from human growth hormone without much side effects. But normal "doping doses" used by athletes are ten to twenty-five international units per day. Essentially, that is five to twenty-five times what one should take for medical use!

Plus, *medical use* would be under a doctor's supervision.

These higher doses can lead not only to hypertension (they can cause fluid retention) but also stroke, even in young athletes. They can also lead to diabetes since it causes glucose breakdown.

This is why anything but very low-dose *legitimate* HGH supplementation should always be through a physician.

Erythropoietin and Adrenocorticotrophin

A hormone that is mainly created by the kidneys, erythropoietin, plays an important role in the body. It stimulates bone marrow to produce red blood cells (erythrocytes). Since red blood cells (RBCs) transport oxygen from the lungs to the rest of the body, an increase in red blood cells can increase stamina for athletes.

But potential side effects for this are significant as well, including hypertension and stroke. Hypertension and stroke are less commonly seen in young athletes since they have very compliant vessels that better tolerate and compensate for hypertension. But other athletes are more susceptible to developing these conditions.

Another possible side effect can be blood cancer. Normally, there may be abnormal cells in the body all the time, but they get corrected by the body on a constant basis. But in addition to stimulating bone marrow, erythropoietin can also stimulate these abnormal cells to grow *before* the body has a chance to repair them. That can lead to cancer.

The other peptide hormone that is abused is *adrenocorticotrophin* (ACTH). Released from the pituitary gland in the brain, this hormone primarily stimulates greater production of cortisol from the adrenal gland. This elevates energy production by increasing the formation of sugar. But if you produce too much sugar and do not use all of it up, this can lead to diabetes and other issues.

Opioids

Opioids are generally safe when taken for a limited time under direction of a physician. However, they are often used in other ways, and opioid use and addiction have created a significant health crisis. Examples of opioids include hydrocodone (Vicodin), oxycodone (OxyContin), fentanyl, codeine, morphine, and many others, including heroin.

Though some people might be puzzled why athletes would abuse opioids, it is not hard to understand. Professional athletes are paid to perform. Yet many get injured. Concerned for their reputation, as well as their team, they want to get back into the game right away. Because they may have recurrent injuries and chronic pain, they start abusing opioids as this stops the pain. But they end up becoming addicted.

Athletes consider themselves strong individuals both physically and mentally, and no doubt many feel they can handle the drug without becoming dependent. But opioids are highly addictive, attaching themselves to specialized proteins in our brain called mu opioid receptors. You may be the most highly disciplined individual and athlete yet can still become addicted. This has become such a serious public health issue that the United States government has aggressively pursued those doctors who too readily have prescribed opioids to patients.

In addition to their addictive qualities, these drugs have numerous side effects, among the most serious being respiratory depression. This causes the body's drive to breathe to go away. The person stops breathing and dies.

Beta2-agonists

Normally prescribed to treat asthma, Beta2-agonists are a group of drugs that open up airways in the body. Some athletes are drawn to using these to open their airways, allowing greater intake of oxygen and better performance.

Yet there are adverse side effects to these as well. Beta2 receptors exist not only in the lungs but also in the heart. These drugs can therefore stimulate the heart, causing palpitations and arrhythmias.

Additional effects from abuse can include headaches, sweats, nausea, and muscle cramps.

Does that mean no athletes are allowed to use these class of drugs? Not necessarily. National and world health organizations do allow these drugs for athletes with asthma. Those athletes benefit from such drugs administered under professional supervision.

Diuretics

Diuretics are drugs that increase the amounts of water and salt expelled out of the body (through urine). These medications are normally prescribed to treat high blood pressure (hypertension) and congestive heart failure.

However, one of the side effects is that diuretics can cause low potassium, which can amplify risks for sudden cardiac death (cardiac arrest). Lesser side effects, due to dehydration, can include muscle cramps, low blood pressure, dizziness, and passing out.

Given their intended use and potential side effects, why would an athlete use diuretics? Sometimes wrestlers and boxers who need to drop weight so they can complete in a lower weight class, find diuretics help lower their (water) weight. Diuretics are also sometimes used to mask other banned drugs. For example, because the diuretic increases the urine volume, this will in turn decrease the *concentration* of the banned drug in the urine and possibly make it less detectable. Also, because of changes in acidity from the diuretic, some drugs may not get excreted (and therefore not detected).

Stimulants

Stimulants have legitimate medical uses, such as for ADHD (attention deficit hyperactivity disorder), narcolepsy (a central brain problem causing extreme tendency to suddenly fall asleep), and obesity (benefitting weight loss).

Yet some athletes are drawn to stimulants, such as amphetamines, as they overactivate metabolism to give greater endurance, power, and speed. Athletes can train longer without getting tired as well as have advantages in competitions.

But these "benefits" come at high cost. Stimulants typically make your heart work harder, aging your heart even more than smoking! In addition, other side effects include insomnia, anxiety, abnormal weight loss, addiction, tremors, and arrhythmias.

Ephedrine, for instance, is a central nervous system stimulant normally employed as treatment for breathing issues, nasal congestion, or low blood pressure. Forms of ephedrine can additionally be found in drugs for ADHD, narcolepsy, and obesity. While the amounts present may be safe for most users, athletes are banned from taking such drugs on the day of competition.

Ephedrine (as pseudoephedrine) can be in nasal decongestants like Sudafed. A significant issue with these drugs surfaced when it was found that some people were acquiring large quantities of Sudafed in order to use the pseudoephedrine as an ingredient in the illegal manufacture of the much more potent stimulants, methamphetamines. The FDA passed new laws requiring that Sudafed no longer be allowed on drugstore shelves but kept behind the counter. Customers now have to show photo ID and stores keep records of buyers for a minimum of two years, with strict limits on how much any individual can buy within a thirty-day period.

Powerful street drugs like amphetamines remain an issue today.

Oddly enough, I recall that when I was an athlete in high school, a stranger approached me after school as I was walking to practice and said, "You want to buy some amphetamines?"

When I told him no, he argued, "Then you're stupid. Why not? They'll let you run and run and never get tired, so you'll be the best player on the field!"

This is how they get you. They find your weakness, your desire to be a star player. Of course, they are not telling you about the side effects.

Even though I was only thirteen, I questioned, "Why would I want to do that? I want my own body to perform. Not some drug to do it for me. That possibly could cause problems and kill me."

Fortunately, even at that young age, I was wise enough to know these drugs were not good for me. Today, we need to educate our young regarding this so they too can brush off those people who want to provide them "magic pills."

Beta-Blockers

A beta-blocker is a medication for high blood pressure, arrhythmias, and to counter tremors. Its function is much the opposite of stimulants.

Given that, which athletes would want to use beta-blockers? Not runners or swimmers or soccer players. It would slow them down. But archers or rifle and pistol target shooters may find use for these substances as they help to give them a steady hand (remember, it counters tremors) and increase accuracy. It does this by lowering heart rate, reducing blood pressure, and calming nerves.

Yet even beta-blockers have side effects as they can make your heart rate and blood pressure too low, cause sleepiness, and even lead to diabetes. The other issue is when someone suddenly stops taking beta-blockers, they can get rebound hypertension and arrhythmias. *Rebound* is the term physicians apply to conditions when they are the result of someone stopping or dramatically lowering dosages of their medication.

Making the Right Choice

The pressures to succeed and best our competitors are intense. Witness the proliferation of private coaches for athletes starting from very young ages.

Abusing performance-boosting medications is an extension of that. But in addition to shifting focus away from the sheer positive pleasures and passions long associated with sporting competition, drug misuse poses risks to health and lives. Some permanent. Sporting organizations have disallowed their use, both to protect players and to level playing fields. Yet other entities seek profits by finding ways to supply illicit medications to competitors.

Ultimately, each player must decide. My hope is that information presented in this book will give athletes plenty of reasons not to manipulate how the body functions and help them understand the high price to be paid for doing so.

CHAPTER 17

RETURNING TO SPORTS

After Diagnosis of Disease

Athletes, like anyone else, can experience disease. But a difference when it comes to serious athletes is that, after they receive a diagnosis, one of the first questions that invariably comes up is "When and how can I return to competitive play?"

Here we will tackle these concerns of competitive athletes. In addition, the latter part of this chapter will address those people participating in recreational sports.

Cardiac Disease

The focus of this chapter will be athletes and cardiac diseases. This will be of special interest to athletes, as not all cardiologists will know those answers about returning to full activity unless they have expertise in competitive sports and cardiac health. This is why, when I became the president of the California chapter of the American College of Cardiology, one of the initiatives I began was *Exercise Health and Sports Cardiology*.

The focus of this mission has been twofold:

- To educate cardiologists in California to better understand sports cardiology and know when they need to refer to experts
- To enhance awareness and importance of exercise health to the general public

Naturally, the correct answer to when an athlete can return to sports will depend on their age, their physical conditioning, and the nature of the cardiac event itself.

Guidelines for determining when athletes can return to competitive play are established through three main sources:

- Bethesda Medical Conference
- American Heart Association Consensus for young patients with genetic cardiovascular disease
- American Heart Association Consensus on master athletes

Note: Master athletes (cited in the third bullet point above) does not signify a level of skill or achievement in some sport. The term master athlete refers to all competitors over the age of forty.

Concern for Aging Athletes

One of the first considerations regarding when and what sports an athlete can participate in again after disease relates to how old they are. Medically, we often group patients by age. For instance, we look at diseases for men under the age of thirty-five differently from those over thirty-five. I will note that some experts in the field choose forty as the dividing line, so here we will say ages thirty-five to forty. For women, the agreed upon boundary number is fifty.

For men over the age of thirty-five to forty and women over the age of fifty, we look at coronary artery disease as the most likely cause of sudden death for those participating in competitive sports. One of the ways in which our body changes over time is that many people get hypertension as they age due to the arteries stiffening. (Stiffening is different from atherosclerosis, which is caused by *blockages* in arteries from fat, etc.) Exercise, healthy diet, maintaining low weight—all these *can* delay the onset of hypertension, though genetics plays a primary role as well.

Anyone in these age groups wanting to do vigorous exercise should have some kind of assessment performed. This would at least include an EKG. If there is anything abnormal in the EKG, an echocardiogram should then be performed. Plus, if the patient has even just one risk factor (such as high blood pressure, high cholesterol, diabetes, family history of coronary disease), they should have a stress test.

There is significant concern for any athlete in these older age groups if there is coronary artery disease or if they have a weakened heart (one with an ejection fraction less than 50 percent, as measured by an echocardiogram).

Such athletes should not participate in any vigorous competitive activity *until* these conditions have been corrected. For instance, if they have coronary disease and we stent the artery, and they only have one blockage, and they go through an appropriate period of rehab while monitoring their condition, and all their numbers return to perfect, then they can return to their activity.

Let me describe various coronary conditions that would pose concern for these athletes by their doctors.

Valve Disease

Valves are the doorways in the heart that allow blood flow to and from the heart chambers. There are four valves in the heart.

Two valves are between the upper and lower chambers, respectively called the tricuspid valve (between right atrium and right ventricle) and the mitral valve (between left atrium and left ventricle).

Of the two other valves, the one that allows blood to pump out of the right ventricle (to the lungs) is the pulmonary valve, while the valve on the left ventricle (allowing blood flow to the rest of the body) is the aortic valve.

The aortic and pulmonary valves each has three leaflets (doors) that open and close. But some people have a congenital condition with only two leaflets in their aortic valve instead of three (we then call this a bicuspid valve—*bi*, meaning "two"). You might never know you have it until detected by an echocardiogram, or we hear a heart murmur (one of the many reasons that doctors use a stethoscope).

Bicuspid valves should function fine from childhood into middle age. But we begin to see issues with this valve after the patient passes fifty. That is because it is not physiologically perfect, and wear and tear over time causes the valve to degenerate. It becomes either tight or leaky. If this condition remains mild, the person can continue competitive sports. But if it becomes moderate or severe, then it must be fixed before they can restart that level of activity.

Aortic Stenosis

Aortic stenosis is when the aortic valve is genetically normal but becomes narrowed. This condition usually does not appear until someone is in their seventies or older. But it could show up in middle age if they had rheumatic fever when they were a child or if they have too much $Lp(a)$, a form of cholesterol that especially tends to cause blockages in arteries. Lp(a) is worse than simply LDL cholesterol, known as "the bad cholesterol." At this point in time, there is no drug that can lower Lp(a) cholesterol.

Doctors will need to determine if a patient's aortic stenosis is considered mild, moderate, or severe.

If someone has mild aortic stenosis, they can do all sports.

With moderate aortic stenosis, someone may do 1A and 1B sports (low-intensity sports, such as golf and bowling, and moderate sports, such as table tennis and volleyball). Examples of categories of different intensity sports are indicated again in the chart below.

With severe stenosis, the patient must not do any sports at all. That is because the valve has become so narrowed that the left ventricle has to pump blood through what is now a very small orifice. There is only a limited amount of output. If the demand goes higher, as it does with exercise, the heart cannot meet it, and the person can pass out.

Fortunately, we can perform surgery to correct for aortic stenosis. While it once was a more invasive open-heart surgery, we now can replace with a new heart valve by going up through an artery in the leg. This has become a common procedure.

So how long should one wait to return to activity after such a surgery? Usually about three months, though it depends on what type of valve they receive and the patient's age and overall health.

In general, if they receive a bioprosthetic valve (made of animal tissue, such as a pig's valve), the patient should be able to do even vigorous exercise after three months.

If they get a mechanical valve, they will need to be on blood thinners for the rest of their life and cannot perform contact sports. But they can do mild exercise after six weeks' recovery and more active exercise like brisk walks and slow jogs after about three months' recovery.

So given its limitations on exercise, why might someone choose a mechanical valve? Because bioprosthetic valves usually last only ten to fifteen years. If the patient is younger, a mechanical valve is generally recommended as they have a much longer lifespan. Of course, with our new through-the-leg approach to replacing a valve, the procedure is much less severe, and a bioprosthetic valve might be a greater consideration.

Aortic Valve with Insufficiency

With this condition, instead of being narrowed (stenotic), the valves do not close well. Much of the blood that is supposed to be pumped out into the body flows *back* into the ventricle (leaky).

Again, if this is mild, the patient can participate in all sports. But once the condition becomes moderate or severe, they should be limited to just 1A sports.

The solution again is to replace the valve, but with severe aortic insufficiency, we cannot do the procedure through the leg. It will require open-heart surgery.

Mitral Valve Prolapse

When the valve between the left upper chamber (atrium) and the left lower chamber (ventricle) closes correctly, blood pumps efficiently out of the left ventricle to the rest of the body with each contraction. But with mitral valve prolapse, the valve's leaflets have thickened and significantly *bulge* (prolapse) back into the left atrium. This can allow some blood to flow backward into the atrium.

It is a fairly common heart condition, and most people do not experience symptoms. If the condition is mild and without symptoms, the athlete can participate in all sports.

But in more severe cases, if this valve leaks severely, if the ejection fraction (measuring ventricle efficiency) has dropped, if there are a lot of PVCs (premature ventricular contractions causing extra heartbeats and disrupting the normal heart rhythm), or there is a positive family history of sudden cardiac death, then we allow no competitive sports at all. Two percent of sudden cardiac deaths in athletes are caused by mitral valve prolapse. There can also be greater risks of blood clots and arrhythmias.

The solution is to replace the valve, and in this case, it again requires open-heart surgery.

Younger Athlete Concerns

Just because an athlete is young and physically fit does not mean there may not be conditions that can affect their participation in competitive sports. Preventing sudden death (cardiac arrest) always remains a focus of doctors for those participating in sports, even with younger athletes.

Here are various conditions that pose particular concern.

Cardiomyopathy (Disease in the Heart Muscle)

Hypertrophic cardiomyopathy is the most common cardiomyopathy in young athletes in the United States. An EKG will diagnose this condition 90 to 95 percent of the time. If it is present, the athlete should not do *any* competitive sports.

Dilated cardiomyopathy is when a virus affects the heart such that the left ventricle becomes dilated, though this can *also* be caused by drug and alcohol abuse. If someone has dilated cardiomyopathy, they absolutely should not be participating in any competitive sports.

Arrhythmogenic right ventricular cardiomyopathy (ARVC) is when the right ventricle (that pumps blood to the lungs) gets infiltrated with fibrofatty tissue rather than muscle, leaving the person at high risk for arrhythmias and sudden death. This condition is present in 2.8 percent of all sudden cardiac death victims in the United States. But in Europe, that number can be as high as 22 percent due to differences in genetic makeup. Someone with ARVC can do 1A activities (golfing, bowling, walking), but clearly not competitive sports.

Myocarditis is an inflammation of the heart muscle that can occur from the flu or certain viruses if you are genetically predisposed to this condition. This affects the heart muscle and its electrical system, causing weakness and negatively affecting the left ventricle's ability to pump. Making this trickier is it can be a transient problem. That is, it can get better or worse (or remain the same). On the other hand, the good news with this condition is that if you retest after six months and the EKG, size of inflammation (determined through blood tests), and echocardiogram are all back to normal, and a twenty-four-hour Holter monitor test shows no arrhythmia, the patient can resume all physical activities again.

Pericarditis is an inflammation of the sac around the heart, which can be induced by virus or infections, radiation, surgery, heart attack, or other illnesses. Symptoms can include chest pain, EKG changes, indications of inflammation (from blood tests), and an echocardiogram showing fluid between the heart muscle wall and the surrounding fat. With this diagnosis, there cannot be any competitive sports. Yet if all testing shows back to normal after six months, the individual can return to all levels of exercise.

Heart Rhythm

Young as well as older athletes often show up to my office after experiencing palpitations (rapid or irregular heartbeats).

Some turn out to be benign rhythm issues that do not impose any limitations on the patient's participation in activities or their capacity. These include the following:

- Sinus bradycardia
- Sinus tachycardia
- Premature atrial contractions or atrial premature complexes (PACs)
- Nonsustained (meaning does not last longer than a few beats) ventricular tachycardia (NSVT)

However, other rhythm issues in athletes do need to be addressed.

AVNRT

Another common rhythm disturbance in athletes is *atrioventricular nodal reentry tachycardia* (AVNRT). This is a disease within the heart's AV node (located at the bottom of the right atrium), which normally sends the electrical signals that make the ventricles contract to pump blood in the body. But AVNRT causes the heart to suddenly beat very fast, up to 220 beats per minute. The patient would certainly feel this!

The good news with AVNRT is that EP (electrophysiology) doctors can use an electrical current created by radio waves (radiofrequency ablation or RFA) to heat the area and cut off the area causing the problem and cure it. After just two to four weeks, the patient can return to all activity without any consequences.

WPW

Another common issue is *Wolff-Parkinson-White* syndrome (WPW). This manifests as palpitations and can cause people to pass out. It shows up as an abnormal EKG. The cause is a short in the electrical pathway from the atrium to the ventricle. This can also be cured with ablation, with the patient returning to full activity after two to four weeks.

Issues with Ventricles

Another area of concern are issues with the heart ventricles, those heart chambers that pump blood either to the lungs or to the rest of the body.

PVCs

Premature ventricular contractions (PVCs) are extra heartbeats that originate in one of the ventricles. A person with PVCs can sense a fluttering or skipped heartbeats in their chest.

After someone is diagnosed with PVCs, if an echocardiogram rules out any structural problems with their heart muscle or severe valve issues, and there is no coronary artery disease (tight blockages of the coronary arteries to the heart), then the person is free to play whatever sports they wish.

However, if someone has very frequent PVCs, meaning more than 20 percent of their beats are PVCs, they probably have some underlying heart condition that is not yet apparent. If we rule out structural heart disease through a cardiac MRI, then we can allow them to participate. In general, if we do not find a reason for frequent PVCs, then they need to be watched closely, since chronic PVCs that are over 20 percent of all beats can lead to cardiomyopathy, which is a weakening of the heart function.

Ventricular Tachycardia

When there are PVCs, but many of the beats are bunched together (a minimum of three PVC heartbeats in a row at a heart rate greater than one hundred beats per minute), then we are now dealing with ventricular tachycardia (VT).

When these PVCs are originating in just one area of the heart and last less than thirty seconds, it is called *nonsustained ventricular tachycardia*. In this case, if we have ruled out structural heart disease and coronary artery disease, then the patient can continue their sports.

On the other hand, if all the PVCs are from only one area of the heart but last longer than thirty seconds, the patient then has *sustained ventricular tachycardia*. This usually indicates some structural heart disease. Still, if a workup finds nothing wrong with the heart muscle or valves, and there is no coronary artery disease, it may be possible that an EP doctor can do ablation. If this cures the condition, the patient can return to full activity after two to four weeks.

However, if the PVC beats are originating from *two* different areas of the heart, this is more dangerous. Medication of beta-blockers should begin and absolutely no competitive sports. This is the sign of a diseased heart, even if we have not yet figured out what that disease is.

Ventricular Fibrillation

Ventricular fibrillation (V-fib) means the heart is quivering rather than pumping blood due to electrical issues in the ventricles. This is a profoundly serious condition that causes sudden death (cardiac arrest), with the patient collapsing since there is no pulse.

If a patient ever experiences this, and even if their heart is successfully shocked so that it resumes function, there will be no more competitive sports for them. They will likely get an *internal defibrillator* (called an implantable cardioverter *defibrillator*, or ICD). The battery-powered ICD detects any irregular heart rhythms and automatically delivers an electric shock so the ventricular fibrillation resumes a normal heartbeat. Once this device is implanted in their body, they can then perform 1A sports after six months.

In general, if someone has an ICD, they should not participate in any competitive sports.

Returning to Recreational Sports and Cardiovascular Disease

Not everyone reading this book will be a competitive athlete, or perhaps they were at one time but now are choosing (or have to choose) more recreational sports as their physical activity. Therefore, I want to speak to what recreational sports would be suitable for people dealing with particular cardiac issues.

We divide recreational sports into three intensities:

- High intensity, such as basketball and soccer
- Moderate intensity, such as doubles tennis, jogging, biking, swimming
- Low intensity, such as bowling, golf, brisk walking

Hypertrophic Cardiomyopathy

If someone has *hypertrophic cardiomyopathy*, they cannot do high-intensity sports. But low- and moderate-intensity sports are fine.

Long QT Syndrome

For a person with *long QT syndrome* (a condition that creates rapid chaotic heartbeats that could cause passing out, a seizure, or in rare cases, sudden death), low- and moderate-intensity recreational sports are fine.

Marfan Syndrome

Marfan syndrome (MFS) is a genetic connective tissue disorder, most commonly in people with long and thin legs and arms (some have wondered if Abraham Lincoln had Marfan). They should only participate in low-intensity recreational sports.

ARVC

Individuals with *arrhythmogenic right ventricular cardiomyopathy* should also only partake in low-intensity recreational sports.

Pacemakers and Internal Defibrillators

Any individual, or any athlete for that matter, no matter if they are young, middle-aged, or older, may end up having pacemakers or defibrillators implanted in them. Those persons also need to know in what sports they can safely participate.

Pacemakers are given to people with *congenital complete heart block*. This is an interruption in the electrical communication between the atriums and ventricles that is present from birth, develops over time, or results out of heart surgery to correct some congenital heart disease in the area close to its electrical system. Pacemakers are also used for those patients with an unusually slow heart rate (bradycardia). A small device surgically placed just beneath the skin of the chest, pacemakers generate electrical pulses to stimulate regular heart contractions.

When a patient is given a pacemaker, that person can resume all activities after about six weeks. But they need to be careful with contact sports, such as football, as that can dislodge the device or dislocate the wire leads in your heart.

Normally, defibrillators are placed in patients that have hypertrophic cardiomyopathy, long QT syndrome, *Brugada syndrome* (rhythm disorder), or ARVC. Electrophysiologists usually put in the ICDs, though as an interventional cardiologist, I place them as well.

Even though the defibrillator was implanted to offset effects of these conditions and protect the patient's life, these patients *should no longer perform high-intensity sports*. The reason is that when we exercise at that level, three things happen: potassium levels increase in our system, our blood becomes more acidic, and there is a surge of catecholamine hormones. When these three things occur with a person who has an implanted defibrillator, the amount of shock needed to convert an arrhythmia back to a normal rhythm goes up. That means they might get shocked, but it may not be sufficient enough to convert a patient out of the arrhythmia.

Now, having said this, research has shown that arrhythmia-caused death in patients who have ICDs is quite rare. One study showed only 1 percent death out of 4,787 patients. So we do not say *don't* exercise. But we do say do not exercise at very high levels. Instead, perform activities like brisk walking so not to raise your heart rate more than 85 percent of your predicted maximum heart rate based on your age. That is also because if your heart rate goes way up, the defibrillator thinks you are having a bad arrhythmia, and you get an inappropriate shock from the defibrillator.

Another reason to avoid high-intensity sports or exercise is they can bring on arrhythmias. Intense exercise with high adrenergic drive (meaning the sympathetic tone is high and it is releasing a lot of stimulating substances such as epinephrine) can cause arrhythmia if the heart has any predisposition to it. When patients incur arrhythmias, even when they are automatically shocked, they might fall and injure themselves (including the possibility of concussions). Certain contact sports can also damage the defibrillator as it is usually implanted just under the skin.

Repetitive motion activities can also pose a high risk to both a pacemaker or defibrillator. Such activities (examples like golf, weight-lifting, swimming, or tennis) can cause *lead fracture*. The lead is the wire attaching the pacemaker or defibrillator to the heart's ventricle. Lead fracture means that wire breaks. Or the lead can be dislodged from its location in the heart due to repetitive motion activities.

The Bottom Line

This chapter has provided general guidance for athletes (or anyone) when returning to physical activity after experiencing heart disease. While there may be limits depending on your circumstances, nearly everyone can resume some form of *ongoing exercise* for your overall health. Armed with this information, *consult with a knowledgeable sports cardiology physician* to determine the right exercise and level of activities for you. This is true even if beginning exercise for the first time and you have heart disease. It is almost never too late to start, and the benefits are impressive.

I want to point out again that while you may have heard of vigorous exercise activities increasing risks for sudden death, this typically occurs with weekend warriors (weekend athletes). Though out of shape, they believe they can jump right into high-intensity activities like basketball or soccer even when their bodies are not used to it. That is a great way to trigger an arrhythmia or heart attack. Plus, these individuals are less likely to have a preparticipation exam from their doctors.

However, a physician health study has shown that *habitual vigorous exercise*, meaning you develop a plan, start slow, and gradually build your level of activity on a daily basis to a high level, can significantly *diminish* your chances of sudden death from exercise. In fact, the study found you can reduce risks of such a catastrophic event *sevenfold* compared to those people who do not exercise regularly at such levels.

What you need to avoid is starting a high-level of exercise when you have not been anywhere near that active. You may like to *think* you are still a twenty-year-old, but you are not (unless you actually happen to be a twenty-year-old).

Ultimately, regular exercise can be good for you as long as it is the *level of exercise that is appropriate for you.*

MOVING FORWARD

You Are In Charge

CHAPTER 18

YOUR HEALTH IS UP TO YOU

Get Moving

Here is a provocative question to consider: "Can I rely entirely on doctors to safeguard my health and well-being?"

We often do. Yet that is not always the wisest path. And another reason that I wrote this book.

All doctors that I interact with always mention diet and exercise to their patients. But I would estimate only 20 percent of doctors *really* push their patients toward diet and exercise, and 80 percent are just trying to manage disease. In good part, this has developed in response to doctors' experiences that most patients will not improve their diet and exercise at the level they need to.

That is, unless something scares the patient, like some major medical event (heart attack, passing out, etc.). Then the person starts thinking, "Now I have to do something about this." All too often, patients come to me *after* some event has occurred. Yet I know in so many cases, such a serious medical crisis could have been avoided entirely. That the person could enjoy a much better, and likely longer, life if they would just be leading a different life.

Change

It is very difficult to change the mentality of people and the culture.

Some attempts at shifting the culture can be seen in the advocacy of modifying certain policies we have become accustomed to, such as removing all soda machines from schools to reduce sugar overload and childhood obesity. There are also new curriculums now at some schools where all able students must run a mile once a week. Some local governments are trying to get our youth to alter their lifestyle by widely implementing these policies at the school level.

Such programs may not only help set the stage for future health habits, there can also be more immediate benefits. Proven benefits of exercise for children include the following:

- Better self-esteem
- Improved concentration and cognitive thinking
- Enhanced overall performance in their education
- Less inclination toward obesity
- Better sleep
- Lower likelihood of being picked on at school

Yet exercising *at any and every age* can be beneficial.

I presently have a patient in his nineties who was a cyclist for many years. He has since given that up and now focuses on brisk walks along with other activities. People who have established routine exercise throughout their life are so often the ones who live a long time.

Closer to home is a cardiovascular surgeon who is eighty-two years old and a lion! Cardiac surgery is very demanding, with the surgeon on their feet for hours at a time to perform precise procedures. He still works from seven in the morning to ten at night without any issues, conducting multiple surgeries daily. He does not bike or jog but has been a mountain hiker all his life, having twice hiked up Mount Everest. Only a few years back, he went up fourteen-thousand-foot Mount Shasta in California. For someone to do that at his age—he is my idol! Turned out that he did end up developing a blockage in his heart and had a stent put in a few years ago. But he is staying active and doing fine without any problems.

These stories and those of many others continue to motivate me both personally and professionally as a physician advising others.

Fortunately, our culture is slowly changing, and there are some positive results. Doctors encouraging exercise and diet is extremely important, but that is just a starting point for the changes that many people need to implement into their lives.

Equally important is we encourage that exercise be done in the proper way for each individual, at whatever level is correct for them. Your general practitioner physician may not have the time, or frankly, the knowledge to advise you on that.

That is why, in addition to possibly finding a sports medicine specialist, that every person at every level of physical fitness should become more educated themselves. Bottom line, it really is up to you. Learn what exercise is right for you. Shift your diet so it supports your body. Find other people leading active lives so you all can support one another. After all, it is your life and your health.

It's your move.

So move!

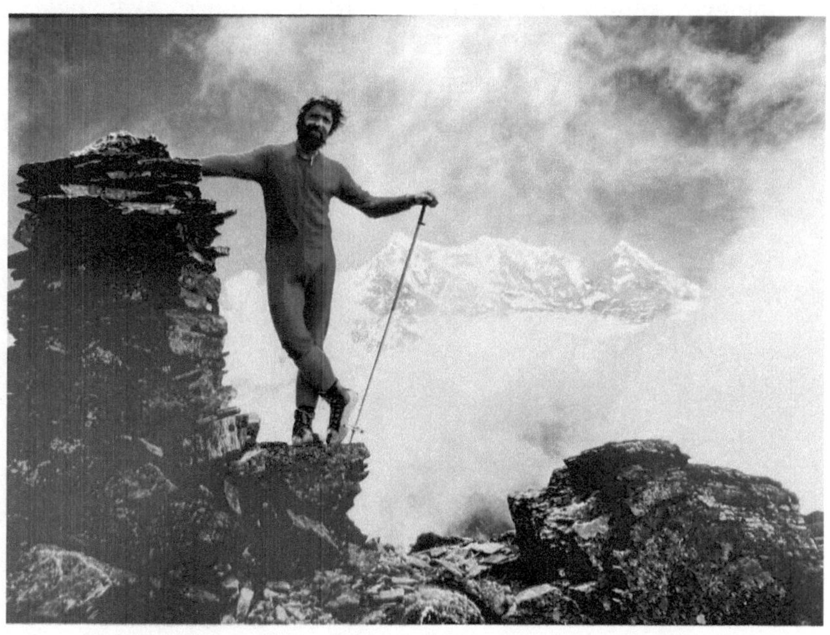

Dr. James Morrissey who is an avid mountain climber still practicing at age 85. Here climbing Mount Everest.

ABOUT THE AUTHOR

Dr. Ramin Manshadi is a practicing Sport Cardiologist, interventional Cardiologist, and the founder and president of Manshadi Heart Institute, inc. He is also the past president of the California Chapter of American College of Cardiology. He is the team cardiologist for Sacramento Republic Professional Soccer team, the director of Soccer Operations for Saint Mary's High School, and sport cardiology consultant for University of Pacific in Stockton, California. He is the cochair and the founder of California Chapter of American College of Cardiology committee on Exercise Health and Sport Cardiology. He is clinical professor at UC Davis Department of Medicine and adjunct professor at Stanford Department of Cardiovascular Medicine. He has authored a book, *The Wisdom of Heart Health*, in the past. He is married and has three children.

www.ingramcontent.com/pod-product-compliance
Lightning Source LLC
Chambersburg PA
CBHW051443250726
48655CB00001B/213